# Pandemic Survival Guide

## How to Survive if You Become Infected

*(Medical Face Masks to Protect Your Family's Immune System)*

**Sandra Santos**

Published By **Bella Frost**

# Sandra Santos

*Pandemic Survival Guide: How to Survive if You Become Infected (Medical Face Masks to Protect Your Family's Immune System)*

**ISBN   978-1-7388267-6-6**

Legal & Disclaimer

suggested remedies, techniques, or information in this book.

Upon using the information contained in this book, you agree to hold harmless the Author from and against any damages, costs, and expenses, including any legal fees potentially resulting from the application of any of the information provided by this guide. This disclaimer applies to any damages or injury caused by the use and application, whether directly or indirectly, of any advice or information presented, whether for breach of contract, tort, negligence, personal injury, criminal intent, or under any other cause of action.

You agree to accept all risks of using the information presented inside this book. You need to consult a professional medical practitioner in order to ensure you are both able and healthy enough to participate in this program.

Table Of Contents

## Chapter 1: Get Your Facts Right

There isn't always any denying that Covid-19 is a life-threatening illness, one which has now restricted us all to the parameters of our houses/global locations and compelled us to lodge to social distancing. It has made us all worry about contracting the virus whenever we have interplay with pals and own family – there may be only a lingering notion of 'what if'.

That said, this pandemic isn't always the give up of the location; we must not deal with it like a lack of lifestyles sentence.

One number one cause why the sickness maintains to scare us to the center is that we do no longer have our statistics proper. Yes, COVID-19 has destroyed the lives of many and made us all live interior, however it isn't the high-quality lethal illness and occurrence in the worldwide right now.

Perspective: Number of Deaths Across the Globe Caused By Different Factors

According to WHO and CDC, Covid-19 has killed over 1.6 million human beings as at December 21 2020.

But consider the fact that:

• Heart sickness kills an predicted 17 million people inside the global and over 655,000 humans in US on my own, each 12 months

• Cancer is projected to kill an expected 606,000 people within the US alone, and over 9 million humans global

• Malaria is expected to kill a child each 30 seconds and over 3,000 youngsters a day, with a worldwide death total of over 2 million human beings

• People die of suicide each 12 months

• Road accidents kill an expected 1.35 million human beings each year!

• Smoking kills an expected 7 million human beings spherical the world.

• And alcoholism kills an estimated three million human beings spherical the area every single three hundred and sixty five days

2

Despite the truth that there are sicknesses that kill a protracted way greater humans than Covid-19, we don't get to pay hobby them masses within the news!

No, this statistics does not reason to spread terror, make you pull your hair out of hysteria, or water down the severity of Covid-19. The nice cause is to help you recognize that at the identical time as the covid-19 is a vital virus that wishes addressing and our interest, you should no longer method it with fear and apprehension.

If you do with the useful resource of hook or via crook agreement the disease, apprehend that eighty one% of its instances are slight, and the price of recuperation is 100% in such instances. Around 14% of cases are slight, and great 5% of the full cases are critical. That only proves that if you do agreement the covid, your opportunities of enhancing from it are excessive.

Some assets have classified COVID-19 deadlier than SARS. However, such property fail to america of the united states that SARS had a

10% fatality rate, even as the fatality price of COVID-19 is less than 2% within the intervening time. Of this, the dying fee of humans under the age of 50 is sincerely over zero.2%.

Mosquitoes kill spherical 2,740 humans almost every day; human beings homicide nearly 1,3 hundred humans in places along side Syria, Palestine, and Kashmir; and 137 people die of snake assaults every day. There are deaths due to one aspect or the alternative every unmarried day, but we are so scared of the covid that many dare now not say its name.

Be Hopeful and Cautious, Not Scared

The covid spreads from one infectious character to any other through breathing droplets. This very reality makes it very contagious – because the droplets simply need to are available in contact together with your eyes, nostril, or mouth to gain entry into your frame. You may also moreover want to pick it up from one of a type surfaces, because it remains on numerous surfaces for special periods.

Luckily, if you undertake the right precautionary measures as directed via fitness officials, you can drastically lessen your probabilities of contracting the virus. It is scary, however it is also avoidable.

While the quantity of deaths because of the covid is growing, so are the instances of healing, as I already said. What we need to recognize is that being scared thru the pandemic will no longer get us anywhere. We want to behave sturdy, added on, wonderful, and hopeful because of the truth that is how we are able to combat our way through this.


Why We Need to Act Positively and Strong inside the Face of Adversity

Here are the motives why we want to behave truly and strongly inside the face of this global adversity.

#: Positivity equals innovativeness

When we're powerful, we start deliberating the exclusive alternatives available to us and search for strategies to fight a trouble.

5

For instance, count on your business enterprise has been notably suffering from the pandemic. In that case, you can best provide you with suitable answers to live on while you are high excellent and may provide you with contemporary survival mechanisms.

#: Apprehension is horrific

Apprehension switches on our strain response, which upsets us extra. Every time you revel in a new name for placed to your gadget, you enjoy stressed out. That triggers your combat or flight response, which produces great physiological changes which encompass rapid respiration, improved heartbeat, and accelerated blood go along with the flow in your muscle agencies and limbs.

Such changes assist you combat the task or danger efficaciously. These changes upward thrust up because of the producing of stress hormones like cortisol. It subsides while the stress hormones lessen, which takes area while you experience as although the risk has ended.

However, if you hold to stay traumatic and worried, like inside the cutting-edge scenario of the COVID-19 pandemic, you could hold having accelerated stages f pressure hormones on your body all of the time. You are probable to live confused for long hours, days, and weeks, that is probable to result in horrible consequences like anxiety, despair and boom your possibilities of affected by sicknesses like immoderate blood stress, diabetes and coronary coronary heart issues.

#: It's better to stay wonderful and satisfied

When you enjoy harassed and disappointed, you fail to well known your blessings. In times of strain, it will become difficult to recognize and recognize first-rate occurrences. That's whilst you slowly draw extra issues in the path of yourself.

You need to be strong, satisfied, and content material cloth because of the reality first-rate then will you have got the ability to tug yourself via this unsettling state of affairs and draw great reviews within the route of you.

Remember the law of enchantment? Like draws like!

If you want unique days to return your manner and in the end step out on the roads, shake arms with people, and absolutely hug your circle of relatives, you need to anticipate undoubtedly. Your wonderful thoughts will do wonders for wonderful and pull tremendous research your manner. For that, you need to stay first-rate and satisfied each day.

#: It's the name of the game to powering thru

Scores of memes get shared every day on social media describing how tough it's far to live with family at domestic. How dull and traumatic it isn't to move anywhere, and the manner hard it's miles for human beings residing very well on my own at home or, worse, of their workplaces. All those memes wonderful growth our anxiety and stress. If we begin to improve our mood and well-being, we're capable of start a series of positivity.

Yes, it is hard to live hopeful and rosy amidst all of the unrest, but it's far plausible.

#: It can assist with productiveness

Most professionals in the meanwhile are running from domestic. Although there's an on-going monetary catastrophe and the professional lives of many people are in jeopardy, a number of us still need to preserve on with our jobs. Working from home is less hard stated than finished, and if we are grumpy, we can not perform the responsibility efficaciously. Taking care of your emotional properly being is vital to make sure you perform well professionally and improve your productivity even in such hard times.

#: It creates a high amazing surroundings

If you're grumpy all of the time, you could make this quarantine tougher on your family individuals quarantined with you. Of route, it is not smooth to smile while there may be fear all round you, but you may do it. If you try to stay tremendous, your positivity will rub off on those human beings you stay with, so you can create a cushty, jovial surroundings as a way to be proper for all and sundry.

For those styles of motives, and the easy fact that it is also higher to be first rate, you want to examine strain control and powerful mood manage in instances of world distress. Once you learn how to do this now, you can pull through any form of impediment and emerge a survivor each single time.

Let us talk about the steps we need to take to make certain that:

## Chapter 2: Accept And Acknowledge Your

## Feelings

To soothe frustration and mitigate chronic pressure, the primary difficulty you need to do is recognize, take delivery of, and widely known your feelings. You are possibly going via a variety of feelings and feelings right now. Many of them can be too chaotic and create a frenzy on your mind. Shunning them or silencing them just received't do the trick.

Your subconscious thoughts is impulsive; it does what you stop it from doing. Think of the way you completed off the whole fudge cake from the fridge each time you knowledgeable your self you have got been on a strict weight loss plan and couldn't consume calorie-wealthy meals. That occurred due to the fact you'd cautioned your self a organization 'no,' and lamentably, your unconscious does no longer sign up 'no,' 'can not,' or 'don't.'

That does not advocate you can't soothe anxiety and put off the strain. You can manipulate tension, uncertainty, and strain, but to do that, you need first of all accepting and acknowledging your feelings.

## The Importance of Accepting and Acknowledging

Accepting your feelings way embracing the fact that you're feeling fine emotions. When you receive some element, you do not question, doubt, or reject its existence. It is much like accepting which you have flu and then going to searching out treatment for it. Every remedy begins offevolved with reputation of the problem. That precept applies to strain and anxiety in uncertain instances as well.

Once you receive that you're feeling pressured out because of all the misery spherical you, you'll understand the foundation reason of your pressure and address it successfully. That will help you renowned it and understand it as part of you.

We are responsible of dealing with pressure within the incorrect way. Instead of soothing ourselves absolutely and embracing our ache, we frequently try to push the feelings deep down with the resource of rejecting them. That is why the pain never ceases; it first-class worsens.

When you get hold of your tension, fears, and pressure, you apprehend there isn't always something to experience embarrassment approximately. You forestall labeling them as horrific or lousy feelings and instead take transport of them as emotions you have to enjoy, and that lets in you to vanish away in case you address them genuinely. Having this method permits you live calm on the identical time as faced via an immoderate emotion, which makes it a lot much less tough so that you can go through it and manipulate it.

How to Accept and Acknowledge Feelings

Here is how you may learn how to acquire and widely recognized your feelings higher so that you can then manage them efficiently.

#: Observe Your Emotions and Feelings

The key to splendor, acknowledgment, and remedy of some thing is keen statement and mindfulness. You need to understand of your feelings and feelings; you need to study them very consciously. Doing this could assist you understand the various symptoms of a particular emotion.

For instance, you can start to pace whilst you experience traumatic, or your tone may additionally turn out to be agitated when you experience forced and irritated due to the disappointment building internal you.

Observe the signs and symptoms and signs and symptoms and signs and signs and symptoms of different feelings, so you understand what results in a selected emotion and might take the right measures to cope with it as it ought to be at the proper time.

Make effective you write the signs and symptoms and symptoms and signs and symptoms of diverse emotions so you can preserve track of them. In a few days, you could get the hold of these signs and symptoms and symptoms and signs and could understand exactly whilst you feel stressful or pressured or indignant.

It is everyday for you, and people spherical you, to experience a choice of numerous feelings, emotions, mind, and reactions consisting of these listed under:

Feeling rather overwhelmed

Feeling emotionally and mentally swamped

Having anxiety and fears wash over you

Racing, disturbing mind that hog your thoughts for hours and days

Sadness and tearfulness

Loss of hobby in recurring sports sports which have been in advance interesting for you

Extreme agitation and restlessness

Feeling helpless and hopeless

Physical signs and symptoms like fatigue, disillusioned stomach, uncomfortable sensations or improved coronary coronary coronary heart price

• Difficulty focusing on easy, ordinary responsibilities

- Difficulty falling asleep and staying asleep at night time time

- Apprehension about being in a public place

- Trouble letting pass of an uncomfortable idea

- Feeling disconnected from cherished ones

- Losing interest in what others say

- Feeling lonely

- Finding it hard to specific your mind to others

- Feeling nobody will understand your fears

- Feeling agitated even as others ask you approximately the manner you enjoy

- Feeling hopeless about your expert scenario

Pay interest to these emotions and write them down. Describe them in element if feasible, and try to offer an cause of each emotion explicitly. Doing this allows you are making a higher enjoy of your emotions and calm your self down.

#: Be Patient with Your Intense Emotion

Once you understand the kind of emotion you experience and additionally come to be aware about its repercussions, excuse your self from the scenario when you revel in that emotion. For example, if you are aware of anger effervescent inner you and also you recognize you can vent out your agitation on a person else, it's miles better to excuse your self from the state of affairs and visit the relaxation room for a couple of minutes.

When you excuse yourself, try to sit someplace peaceful and quiet to allow the emotion take its time interior you and subside on its private. Whatever emotion you feel, be it tension, worry, frustration, disappointment, anger, or a aggregate of lots of those, it'll first upward push to its top and then very little by little reduce substantial.

It typically takes an emotion 12 minutes to gather its pinnacle and then fade away. That way if you do now not react to intense emotions and do not keep without delay to them, they will reduce great with out you having to do some component to control them.

Whenever you experience:

• Exhausted due to the fact you've got been searching after your youngsters all day prolonged

• Sad due to the fact you absolutely heard the statistics of any other loss of life due to Covid-19 in your location

• Angry because you have to finish your gadget-associated duties and your circle of relatives isn't assisting with own family chores,

Excuse your self from the scenario; bypass someplace non violent, and take a look at your emotion patiently.

#: Take Deep Breaths

When it's far honestly you and your emotion, take sluggish, calming breaths and feature a have a examine the emotion as you inhale and exhale. You can also additionally need to yell at your youngster, pound your fist on the desk, run away, or get right right into a heated argument together with your associate. These are all the precise reactive thoughts your excessive emotion creates indoors you.

Acknowledge them patiently and allow the extreme emotion bubble.

Keep searching at it and the manner it makes you sense. If you have were given had been given the strength to put in writing about it right now, do so, but if it feels difficult to select up a pen or take notes for your cellphone/laptop, try this later; for now, lightly watch the emotion. Give it a few minutes; it's going to fade out.

#: Avoid Labeling

During this time of calm observation, you could get a robust urge to label your emotions and feelings. Sadly, that is how most mother and father assume at some point of our existence. We address anger as horrible and horrific, a few issue of which we must be concerned.

The fact is this, even though:

Our belief of factors and our reaction is what makes something true or horrible. Every emotion teaches you something approximately yourself and is a response to a situation you have were given have been given been in; if you harness your emotions constructively, they will pleasant help you reply higher to feelings.

Whether you are rather agitated or swamped or seething with anger, recognize it as a mere emotion. Avoid tagging on labels. The minute you prevent seeing a few detail as a awful issue, it diminishes tremendous.

#: Accept How You Feel

After a few minutes of this conscious, gentle remark, you can experience a non violent discount in that emotion's depth. If earlier you felt intensely agitated, it'd have reduced to moderate annoyance. If you were fuming with anger, it'd have changed to moderate pressure.

At this element, gain how you revel in and engage in a relaxed speak with that emotion. For example, in case you felt a aggregate of fear and agitation because of the discovery of 10 more covid instances for your area and the truth that you have not been capable of visit your mother and father residing streets down because of the pandemic, get hold of that you are feeling indignant and unhappy.

Verbal acknowledgment of your emotions permits you take shipping of and soothe them better. You ought to say a few difficulty like, 'I experience irritated and unhappy due to the pandemic that has affected my habitual lifestyles' or 'I am careworn because I fear my circle of relatives and I may additionally agreement the covid.' It also can moreover even revel in scary and overwhelming to blurt out the manner you enjoy verbally, but announcing it aloud permits release the built-up anxiety internal you, so permit it's miles.

It is k if, at this detail, you enjoy like crying or perhaps yelling. You are to your very very own, and there may be no damage in venting out the frustration. Writing about it's far a few different manner that allows many humans to make peace with the unsettling feelings inner them. Do whatever feels proper to you and allow your emotions pour out.

You then need to have interaction in a peaceful talk in conjunction with your emotion. If it rattles internal, ask your self why you enjoy that manner. If you sense as even though now not anything will ever be proper, recall why you experience that manner. Doing this permits you dig out the foundation motives of your intense, unsettling emotions. Jot down the information so you can mirror on it to recognize your emotions better.

#: Identify the Triggers

Moreover, attempt to dig out and discover what triggers those feelings. You can be disappointed about the scenario typical, together with the quarantine, however what exactly came about a couple of minutes within the past that made you lose your calm? Was it the reality that you wakened late, had to make breakfast for your circle of relatives, and flip in a file in an hour? Or were you upset because of the reality you have got were given been living at your place of business for the past one week and haven't been capable of cross once more on your associate at home, and seeing a message from him heightened your misery?

Identifying the triggers helps you figure out the notable situations, events, and topics that exacerbate your pressure so you can then locate likely and effective strategies to manipulate them.

This will be noted in next chapters.

For now, you need to behave patiently and lightly at the aspect of your severe emotions on every occasion you enjoy them. Moreover, train your youngsters, family, roommates, or whosoever you are sharing the space with these days to do the equal.

If you aren't on my own in this quarantine, it becomes even tougher to manipulate your emotions because of the reality you may without issues pick up stress and unrest from someone else. Helping others receive and broadly recognized their feelings make matters simpler for everybody.

If you determine on those measures for some days, you may brief have a better hold of your feelings. Meanwhile, educate yourself to speak simply to yourself and others because of the truth powerful phrases calm severe feelings and create greater calming feelings internal you.

The subsequent economic damage talks a bit more approximately this:

To Act Positive, Think Positively

Every time adversities assault us, we lose our calm, and our mind is going berserk. Usually, the mind that pop into the thoughts first in such occasions are narrow, terrible, and reactive.

When you heard approximately the coronavirus outbreak to your america of the us, you probable thought of approaches it'd take over the whole u.S. Of the united states and your united states of america. You may moreover have involved about your survival similarly to your family's survival. You also can have grow to be panicky and may without a doubt have entered into an severe argument with a loved one.

While it's miles regular to experience and react this manner beneath such unsettling and frightening conditions, in case you preserve thinking and behaving on this way, you will most effective lose your sanity. You turns into more of a stress cooker whistling and blowing off steam thru lousy measures now after which. That is not a healthful method to life and takes a toll in your intellectual and emotional fitness.

To manage your mood efficaciously so you live as high-quality as viable to spread that optimism round, educate yourself to count on absolutely, and construct a growth-oriented mind-set. When you sense exquisite, your moves emerge as significant and positive too.

How to Think and Act Positively

Here is how you may do that.

#: Acknowledge Your Disturbing Thoughts

Just as you stated your excessive emotions as a way to make peace with them, renowned your disturbing and erratic thoughts so that you calm them gently. We regularly shun our undesirable thoughts and push them within the back of our minds in hopes of having rid of them. Doing that does more damage than accurate and exacerbates such mind in place of removing them.

To bring together a tremendous mind-set, renowned annoying mind in addition to the emotions they stir. If you fear you could agreement COVID-19, write that notion down. If you observed the sector goes to stop, positioned that down to your magazine. Whatever fears, troubles, and negativities pop to your head, jot them down on your mag.

Thank your mind for bringing the ones thoughts to your interest. Additionally, avoid labeling them. Simply take shipping of them as issues which may be bobbing up due to the cutting-edge situation.

#: Question the Genuineness of Your Fears and Worries

Once you have acquainted and mentioned some of your worrying mind, question their authenticity. Most of our fears are mere ramifications of our minds; they do not maintain any truth.

Nonetheless, we take transport of and do not forget them, this is why they wreak havoc in our minds. To be satisfied, we need to create uplifting and healthful ideals. That can get up if we do away with poisonous thoughts from our minds as a manner to make extra room for greater wholesome ideals.

A right manner to do this is to impeach the genuineness of your unconstructive and toxic mind. Many such thoughts are mere fears and issues; they will be no longer huge. When you recognise that, it will become much less complex to discard them from your thoughts for appropriate.

Here is how you can do that.

• Take one fear or debilitating trouble at a time and reflect on it.

• If you notion, 'I may additionally settlement the covid and die,' consider how true this belief is and whether or no longer or not there's actual records to manual this idea.

• Examine your adventure records. Look for the signs and signs and symptoms and symptoms of covid which encompass dry cough, immoderate fever, shortness of breath and fatigue.

• Similarly, examine each frightening idea you've got got to research its authenticity. Some fears, which include the ones related to the spread of the virus to your area, might also have valid evidence. In such instances, recognize which you have not any manipulate over this case, however you could manipulate your self and encourage the ones round you to have a take a look at precautions. If you do this, you have were given accomplished your thing in stopping the disorder from spreading.

• As for exceptional concerned thoughts, take transport of the fact that fears and problems are part of our lifestyles and could live with us no matter what. We can't prevent such worries genuinely, however we're able to pick to reply to them actually.

• If you've got acquainted and acknowledged such mind and understood how some of them aren't real, you need to live calm and update such thoughts with uplifting ones.

#: Find Positive Replacements for Unsettling Thoughts

Whatever perception disturbed you, trade it to some thing extra excessive great and motivating. If you concept, 'We will live in quarantine for the complete yr now, and nothing receives again to normal,' trade it to some thing greater realistically brilliant.

For example, you may say, 'This quarantine might be over speedy, and we are able to fast bypass over again to our everyday existence.' You also can say, 'researchers have already created numerous vaccines for COVID-19. All the distress will surrender quickly — I actually want to apprehend in there."

Use this approach with all your frightening thoughts so that you can exchange them to greater exceptional ones. Your mind have an effect in your temper and attitude that then shapes your behavior and movements. When you feed your mind notable thoughts, it creates more mind in the direction, which allows you feel incredible at some degree in the day.

Every time you turn on any records channel and find out about each exceptional provoking coronavirus statistics, or experience agitated about how social distancing has ruined your social life, take deep breaths, well known your frightening mind and update them with extra uplifting ones.

#: Practice Positive Affirmations Throughout the Day

Additionally, exercising extremely good affirmations targeted on peace, happiness, tranquility, positivity, abundance, prosperity, and actual fitness at some degree in the day. Affirmations are effective pointers you repeat generally over verbally or in written form, or every, as a way to verify them for your thoughts.

Affirming a proposal to your subconscious mind approach making your subconscious mind gather some thing because the reality. That takes region even as you repeat the concept regularly. Doing this makes your subconscious recognize the concept as a few element vital to you in order that it then includes it for your belief tool.

That perception then makes you observed in a comparable course, which helps you create more terrific thoughts that circulate out in the universe and draw excellent evaluations your manner.

To stay glad, enjoy peaceful, and fight the covid pandemic with suitable fitness and cheer, create affirmations on the ones factors and exercise them at a few level within the day.

Here is how you can try this:

• Make quick, easy, and top notch affirmations associated with health, happiness, peace, particular well being, and the likes.

• Ensure the affirmation has splendid terms handiest by using the use of manner of casting off any phrases with a horrible connotation together with 'no,' 'now not,' 'by no means,' and 'can't' from the belief. Your subconscious can't apprehend such phrases; it omits them from suggestions to reframe them for that reason. If you chant, 'I will no longer contract the illness' or 'I will no longer be sad,' your subconscious will skip over the 'no longer' from those tips and change them to, 'I will settlement the virus' or 'I may be sad.' Positive hints help rewire your mind to assume with a bit of fulfillment and draw better research and possibilities your way.

• Keep the confirmation present-oriented, this means that that it ought to recommend that you have attained what you're chanting. Instead of chanting a future-oriented concept at the side of, 'I may be healthful,' create a gift-orientated one at the side of 'I am healthful.' This way, you popularity your subconscious on manifesting your desires within the gift 2d.

• Once your affirmation is ready, chant it aloud or maybe write it down slowly and consciously. Pay interest to each phrase as you utter it and allow the vibration ring in your ears. Focusing at the brilliant confirmation by myself soothes your racing thoughts because it diverts your interest from all of the chaotic thoughts wreaking havoc internal it to that peaceful idea.

• As you chant it, near your eyes and be given as true with your self in that state of affairs. If you are chanting how satisfied you experience, take delivery of as true with being your happiest self. If you're declaring a health-primarily based truely affirmation, visualize your self feeling emotionally and bodily wholesome. Doing this facilitates prompt the RAS (Reticular Activating System) of your mind and makes it cognizance higher on the respective thought. The RAS is a region for your brain that filters out useless facts so you can popularity better at the important statistics. It gauges the importance of various quantities of information for you via reading your diploma of reputation and interest to them. When you chant a wonderful concept time and again, confirm it for your mind and visualize it, the RAS perceives it as important. It then saves it in your lengthy-time period reminiscence, which lets in you attention on it better.

• Make certain to visualize, chant, and write pleasant affirmations based totally on everyday obligations and the popular improvements you choice to bring in your temper, fitness, personality, and lifestyles day by day, so one assist you to stay content, calm, and satisfied.

Here are a few useful affirmations initially:

I am wholesome and satisfied.

I enjoy glad and non violent about my life.

I inhale peace and exhale strain.

I spread positivity all spherical me.

I draw exquisite testimonies inside the direction of me.

I am a deliver of comfort for people round me.

I am powerful, centered, and satisfied.

My expert lifestyles is going properly.

I am active and live a satisfied, lively way of life.

I am content cloth material with my life.

#: Slowly undertake a Growth Mindset

If you do all the above frequently, you may slowly assemble a greater remarkable attitude as a way to inspire you to think hopefully during hard times. You now need to work on it further in order that it will become extra growth-orientated.

A boom-orientated mind-set is one that makes you enjoy hopeful and nice approximately yourself and your existence. It permits you recognize that expertise and capability can constantly expand, and you can continuously turn out to be a higher model of themselves.

On the alternative hand, a set or proscribing mind-set is the as an alternative conservative counterpart of a boom mind-set that makes you revel in that your know-how can't develop past a positive point. Since you experience your growth constrained, you accept as true with you studied conservatively underneath difficult times and can awareness on exceptional the worst-case situation.

Unfortunately, the pandemic situation the sector is experiencing has triggered lots of us to nurture a limiting mind-set. We worry the worst very last results of any information we get, it's far why it turns into hard for us to be hopeful of a better day after today. To assemble a increase mindset, work at the strategies said above, and add the subsequent for your positivity regimen:

• Add phrases like "however", "however", and "now" to your speech. Such phrases offer you with need that at the identical time as you cannot understand the manner to do a little factor or are but to attain a positive final consequences, there is desire that you may do it inside the destiny. For instance, as opposed to pronouncing, 'I can not draw,' say, 'I cannot draw but,' or alternate statements like, 'There is not any vaccine for covid in my location' to 'There isn't any vaccine for covid in my location, but.' Making this variation makes your speech greater great and your thoughts-set greater boom-orientated.

• Pay interest to yourself-speak, it truly is the manner you talk to yourself. If you are harsh with yourself on every occasion you're making a mistake, or assume negatively, or lose your calm, or reflect onconsideration on doing something ambitious, your self-speak might be bad. Examples of this encompass, 'I am in no manner going to be satisfied,' 'I am horrible at

Statistics,' 'Today goes to be but some other terrible day' and the likes. Change your self-talk from poor to remarkable by using acknowledging such mind and changing them with high-quality substitutes.

• Create a plan to do your responsibilities and set milestones for them. If you want to make spaghetti with meatballs, create a time desk for it. If you have got got to finish a weblog-positioned up for a purchaser, plan therefore. When you slowly gain small milestones and note your self progressing with responsibilities, you revel in first-rate about yourself. This excessive first rate feeling breeds a boom-oriented thoughts-set that enables you nurture fantastic thoughts.

Additionally, ensure to consider your benefits to nurture gratitude.

#: Be Grateful to Nurture Gratitude

Gratitude fuels positivity, and happiness. The minute you depend even one in each of your blessings or reflect onconsideration on a unmarried aspect that gives comfort and comfort in your existence, you right away sense higher. Your mood brightens up, and anxiety-ranges lower extensive. The uncertain times we're all living in require us to be greater content material fabric and thankful.

Many oldsters are complaining about how this quarantine time is a punishment, the manner it has made us simply stagnant, and the manner it has interfered with the satisfactory great of our life.

Undoubtedly, it has modified our ordinary lifestyles and is hard to deal with, but if we stop perceiving it as a death sentence and attention on what we are capable of study, we're capable of enjoy higher. Doing this helps us make higher use of this time, understand it as an possibility and improve our mood.

To do this and to nurture gratitude in standard, try the following recommendations:

• Upon waking up each morning, reflect onconsideration on one element that looks as if a blessing. You have to thank the universe or some thing strength you accept as true with in for supplying you with a new day to stay. You is probably thankful for being healthy, waking up feeling glowing, sleeping on a cushty bed and some thing else you consider you studied is a blessing.

• After each three hours, bear in thoughts one component that makes your life better, at the side of the capacity to paintings, a system that can pay nicely, having a own family with the resource of your aspect, having sufficient cash to shop for food, and so forth.

• It is higher if you could jot down your benefits and replicate on their significance for a couple of minutes; this may help you feel higher.

• Think of those disadvantaged of the advantages you have were given and are residing in a long way more tough situations compared to yours.

• Every day, take five minutes to discover at least 3 positives about the quarantine scenario. That does now not suggest you need to understand the covid as an incredible hassle. Of direction, it's far lifestyles-altering, however if you preserve seeing the situation it has created as some component 'lousy,' you may handiest experience gloomier and further annoyed. You can be grateful for things which includes:

Getting a harm from an otherwise worrying recurring.

Not having to power to paintings each day for a while, which permits you relax more.

Getting greater time to mirror on yourself.

Having greater time to spend along with your youngsters.

Not meeting too many humans and getting time to lighten up. That is mainly a huge gain for introverts who select out up at the electricity of others in social conditions.

Getting a harm out of your academic lifestyles and obligations.

Getting greater time to observe your preferred books, pay attention on your preferred music, and spend time doing sports sports which you could not locate time for in any other case, collectively with portray, dancing, pottery, and plenty of others.

Work on these recommendations every day; in multiple days, in place of despair, you may experience hopeful.

#: Talk Politely and Positively with those Around You

In addition to being powerful and type to your self, do the equal with those spherical you. Whether you are speaking for your 5-three hundred and sixty five days-vintage son or your 27-12 months-vintage cousin who came to visit from each other u.S., and is now quarantined with you, your boss through Skype, or every body else, accomplish that politely.

It is easier to be worked up nowadays, even supposing the slightest of things cross incorrect. Your kid cries, and you revel in like yelling at him. Your sibling drops a plate, and also you lose your calm. Your boss receives agitated at you for turning in an challenge late, and you enjoy like screaming at him thru the Skype call. This is understandable. However, in case you hold with this conduct and supply into your maddening urges each time, you will nice end up emotionally risky.

To enhance the way you experience, communicate lightly, gently, and courteously with absolutely everyone round you.

• If someone says a few thing scary, take deep breaths or excuse yourself from the scenario to sit back out your frustration. Once you experience higher, offer an purpose in the back of the state of affairs to him/her politely.

• If you phrase someone feeling unhappy, raise up his/her spirits with the resource of announcing type topics to him/her.

• Appreciate people for their developments and strengths. Doing this brightens up their temper, and at the same time as you observe someone smiling because of you, you enjoy higher approximately yourself.

• Greet humans well each time you talk to them, be it bodily or without a doubt.

• Give people want each time they point out the miserable state of affairs. Talk to them approximately the contemporary-day records, information, and figures, and communicate the only-of-a-type prevention measures inquisitive about the useful aid of your usa's government and authorities to keep the situation under manage.

If you often artwork on a number of those measures, you can enjoy higher and more excessive pleasant from inner; your demeanor may encourage others to sense the equal. As you look at the above measures, you moreover may additionally want to art work on keeping an powerful everyday so you carry out your habitual obligations well.

Let us find out the manner to try this within the subsequent step.

## Chapter 3: Maintain A Consistent Routine

Stress and tension often come from now not having a steady recurring and from feeling chaotic. If you awaken within the afternoon day by day and go to bed at dawn without getting something meaningful completed in among that duration, you're probable to experience pressured and stressful.

In this time of social distancing and quarantine, masses humans have resorted to a unusual routine, one that super revolves round binge-searching films on Netflix, staying on social media for hours on give up, and doing not anything effective. While this is all right for a day or , turning the ones sports activities proper proper into a recurring makes existence monotonous, worrying, and worrying.

Being in quarantine does no longer mean you cannot carry out your routine activities or live calm and happy. It only method you stay in, restrict bodily interplay, and maintain social distancing. You can despite the fact that do many stuff you probably did formerly. When you preserve yourself busy in certainly one of a kind sports activities, you do now not offer your thoughts enough time to get lost to darkish, gloomy places. Instead, you live first rate and glad.

Moreover, having a ordinary enables you complete extra responsibilities on time; it improves your productiveness and permits you manipulate time effectively. Additionally, it makes you enjoy sane due to the fact at the same time as you are occupied and engaged in obligations, you do not revel in that life has bogged down or has grow to be annoying.

How to Create a Healthy Routine

Here is how you could have a wholesome recurring on this quarantine.

#: Build a Proper Sleep and Rising Routine

Start thru developing with a snooze recurring. It seems amusing to sleep overdue and sleep in all day prolonged, however whilst this becomes a regular, lethargy and monotony creep to your life. To have a healthful recurring throughout the day, first assemble a right sleep and developing normal.

Based at the massive kind of hours you need to sleep at night time (among 7 and 9 hours for adults), set your sleep time and developing time accordingly. Go to mattress and wake up on the set times, even if you hold tossing and turning for a few nights. Soon, you'll modify to this routine and sleep properly.

#: Maintain Fixed Meal Times

Try to have fixed and proper mealtimes. Do no longer skip breakfast; alternatively, make sure you have got a healthful one. Have lunch around midday with a snack inside the afternoon, and have dinner three hours earlier than your bedtime. This everyday ensures you enjoy glowing and lively and perform your routine duties actively.

#: Create a Schedule for Routine Academic and Professional Activities

Whatever expert and educational duties you have got got, set a time desk for them and work because of this. Treat your art work and studies such as you possibly did even as you had to go to the administrative center or college/university. If your artwork hours have been from 9 am to 5 pm, paintings on your professional responsibilities at some degree in the identical period. If you have online lessons nowadays, take them on time, and when you have any assignments/initiatives to paintings on, accomplish that eventually of your regular class hours. Adopting this technique permits you whole crucial duties on time and feature a few issue widespread to do at some stage inside the day.

#: Stay Clean and Fresh

Do no longer forget to take a tub, ideally a heat bathe each day. Wash your arms at some point of the day; sanitize your hands, and disinfect your whole domestic.

#: Spend Time with Family

Spend time with own family and cherished ones, and stay connected to them irrespective of being restrained to your own home/workplace.

Here is how you can do that:

• If your family are away, ship them a message each day.

• Use social media to stay up to date with pals.

• Call your circle of relatives, one relative/friend a day and find out how they're doing

• If you have got got own family contributors staying with you, spend an hour or two of brilliant time with them over a meal or in any other case each day.

• You can also need to play board video video games or unique video video games with cherished ones to have fun collectively.

Make own family time part of your every day ordinary so you revel in emotionally calm.

#: Exercise

Additionally, make some room for exercising in your ordinary because it allows you stay healthy, active, and satisfied. It improves the producing of temper-enhancing hormones on the side of dopamine and serotonin, which keep you enthusiastic, confident, and glad.

Now which you have greater loose time, use it appropriately thru doing a rigorous physical hobby each day. Start through doing a little element complete of existence which embody aerobics, yoga, dancing, or a aggregate of these for 10 mins and slowly growth the period to 1/2 of-hour. In a few days, you may experience extra energized and high quality than in advance than.

In addition to having a healthy, regular routine, add more tremendous sports sports to your routine to make it calming and to combat pressure higher.


Incorporate Healthy Activities in Your Routine and Enjoy

Stress and tension certainly exit your existence on the same time as you've got interplay in vast, pleasant sports activities activities. Now that you do now not need to circulate back and forth from side to side from art work each day, and on account that you've got greater time at your disposal, upload the subsequent widespread sports into your normal so that you can relax:

#: Read Books

Ensure which you observe at the least ten pages of an extremely good ebook, especially one on self-development or any place of interest you experience each day. Although this dependancy takes a most of half of-hour, it leaves you feeling fantastic.

#: Listen to Podcasts

Use Google to look for exciting podcasts related to your chosen problem be counted and spend an hour or taking note of them each day. If they'll be on self-improvement, make sure to put into effect the strategies referred to inside the podcasts.

#: Learn New Skills

Many human beings are complaining approximately how they've got not anything to do throughout this time. What we don't comprehend is that nature has given us the existing of time that we are able to located to accurate use through reading new talents. Find a few abilties you've got desired to look at for pretty a while, find tutorials online, and art work on them regularly.

Spare an hour or to learn how to do picture designing, internet development, weblog writing, knitting, pottery, painting, or a few other ability you need to feature on your skillset and diversify it. Keep your expert dreams in mind and have a look at a talent or two pertinent to them simply so while you resume your proper work-existence after the quarantine is over, you display your mettle to all people.

#: Meditate

Meditation is a surefire manner to loosen up your compelled nerves and mitigate tension. It allows you recognition at the prevailing moment and soothe your racing mind. While there are various meditative techniques, a easy one for novices is as illustrated underneath:

• Sit with out a trouble on the floor, yoga mat, or the couch, and near your eyes.

• Inhale thru your nose at your everyday pace and watch your breath input your frame and flow into.

• Exhale via your mouth and lightly take a look at your breath because it exits your frame.

• Keep respiratory like this for two minutes and be aware about the precise sensations internal your body.

• When you wander off in concept, bring your attention again in your breath, and gently check it. It will take you some attempts to get the grasp of it, however speedy, you may.

In best 2 minutes, you will revel in greater snug than earlier than and will enjoy clarity of thoughts as nicely. Practice this exercise at least twice a day and slowly increase the duration to 5 mins in keeping with consultation. Carry it out regularly and mainly every time you sense pressured. Soon, you may have better manipulate of your mind, mood swings, and sadness.

#: Spread Awareness approximately COVID-19

Do your element in spreading popularity approximately Covid-19, the manner to prevent it and create reputation around the to be had vaccines amongst humans to your social circle via textual content messages, pictures, and emails via online systems and system. Doing this makes you sense correct approximately yourself for doing some component high-quality and decreases your pressure.

#: Have Fun

Take out time to do some thing a laugh and enjoyable for an hour every day. You may want to observe a movie, Snapchat with pals, interact in position-gambling with children, or do whatever else that permits you unwind and feature a laugh.

Also, live linked and up to date with the present day-day-day affairs and contemporary discoveries on covid19, but try not to allow the horrifying information mess together with your head. Stay hopeful and amazing; higher times will come sooner than you determined.

## Chapter 4: What Is A Pandemic?

A pandemic is the global spread of a modern disease2. A pandemic takes place at the same time as a brand new infectious disorder emerges and spreads around the arena, and maximum human beings do not have immunity. Viruses that have brought on beyond pandemics are stated to normally originate from animal viruses. Viruses that skip from animal to human beings are known as Zoonosis viruses.

Some elements of pandemic can seem just like seasonal influenza at the same time as other tendencies may be quite remarkable. For instance, most pandemics have an impact at the respiration gadget and influenza can motive infections becoming pneumonia. While those ailments can have an effect on all age groups, it generally impacts more youthful kids and the aged the most. Many instances can bring about confined infection in which the man or woman recovers completely without remedy. However, intense instances upward push up most typically in humans having a whole lot of preceding medical situations.

For many illnesses, the complete quantity of individuals who get extensively unwell can range. However, the effect or severity has a tendency to be better in pandemics in element due to the a wonderful deal larger form of people in the populace who lack pre-gift immunity to the ultra-cutting-edge illness. When a huge a part of the population is inflamed, despite the fact that the proportion of these infected that go straight away to boom extreme disease is small, the whole type of excessive times may be quite huge.

For maximum pandemics, the high-quality stages of hobby is probably predicted to occur inside the popular influenza season duration for a place. This is probably inside the temperate weather zones for wintry weather months, for example. This is idea to be from each the close to quarters humans percentage in the direction of winter months and due to the reality viruses and micro organism continue to exist outside of the body for shorter periods of time in warmer temperatures.

An extra detail no longer previously seen inside the phrase is the near proximity of humans residing close to one another. More human beings stay in cities and further metropolis regions than ever in advance than in human information. This close proximity makes it simpler for contagious illnesses to spread.

How Pandemics Spread

Several elements weigh in on how contagious an endemic or bacteria can be. The longer the infectious duration of a ailment, the higher the chance to infect others. The longer bacteria can live outside of the frame, the extra the opportunities someone comes into touch with it. Hygiene, sanitation, and get entry to to clean water also can effect the charge at which a plague spreads.

If a ailment doesn't display signs or signs and symptoms and symptoms for an extended time frame, then it's miles much more likely the inflamed character will come into contact with greater people increasing the probabilities to infect others. If a virulent disease or bacteria lasts a long term out of doors of the frame, then it is also much less tough to bypass from individual to unsuspecting character.

Spreading Through Contact

Viruses and Bacteria are with out problem unfold despite the fact that moving into touch with each of them and then transferring them into your frame by means of touching your face, for example. They live and reproduce inside the frame after which leave the frame via fluids. These fluids can be saliva, mucus, tears, urine, feces, or even blood. Because bacteria and viruses are so small, they high-quality want the most minute quantities of fluids to adventure.

Both may be unfold via ingesting undercooked or unwashed meals. This isn't always unusual in restaurants or possibly complete groups wherein washing meals and handwashing isn't popular.

Areas with customs that involve touching others, which encompass handshaking, hugging, and kissing can see epidemic like spreads of infection. Since those customs are so ingrained inside the population, infectious illnesses typically get a big head begin of infecting humans in advance than they're located.

Viruses and bacteria are frequently decided on typically touched gadgets in high website site visitors areas. Doorknobs, rest room surfaces, countertops, and masses of others are all places in which humans grow to be inflamed with small germ debris.

Germs are results unfold from man or woman to person, from character to item or from object to character. No touch is steady in a pandemic. Increased hygiene and ordinary cleansing of surfaces is critical.

Spreading Through Exchange of Bodily Fluids

Similarly to contact spreading, the direct sharing of physical fluids can transmit infectious sickness. Kissing, sexual touch, sharing cups and utensils, sharing meals, sneezing, coughing, or perhaps being gift on the equal time as someone else is the usage of the restroom are approaches to unfold germs.

While a number of the ones are intentional, a few are not.

Purposeful contact with others is usually risky throughout a virulent disease. Because humans can be infections without showing signs and symptoms, there can be constantly the possibility that someone has a contagious sickness unknowingly.

Accidental touch with bodily fluids from a person else is pretty common and regularly innocent. In a virulent disease however, it's far risky and to be prevented. Sneezing, coughing, or maybe being present at the same time as someone else is using the restroom are presumed accidental strategies of spreading germs. Always use warning in public settings.

Spreading Through the Air

As previously stated, sneezing, coughing, or maybe being present while someone else is the use of the restroom are approaches to spread infectious illnesses. These are recounted strategies of airborne transmission.

Droplet

The fluids leaving the body, that aren't in massive hundreds, are referred to as droplets. These droplets are very small and depart the body while coughing, sneezing, the use of the restroom, or even truly respiratory. Because droplets are generally nonetheless huge sufficient to be pulled down via manner of gravity pretty speedy, they aren't seen to be a real "airborne" chance through many agencies. However, droplet spreading is taken into consideration airborne withing about 6 toes, or meters, from the supply (inflamed character).

Because they do deliver manner to services and rest on them, they may be the number one supply of touch spreading.

Aerosol

When droplets are so small they end up suspended inside the air for extra intervals of time they're considered to be Aerosols. Aerosols can be carried with the aid of a breeze, air waft systems, fans, and may be suspended in air lengthy sufficient for humans to pass thru them. These smaller particles can journey lots similarly than droplets and it isn't unusual to concentrate of room to room transmission thru air go together with the drift. Because the size of aerosols is an lousy lot smaller than droplets, air filtration is normally a trendy on the equal time as preventing germs spread this manner.

## Warding Off Germs and Infection

The superb way to prevent from being inflamed with the resource of a deadly disease or bacteria is to keep away from it altogether. That approach fending off humans. Since people are the supply of spreading germs, averting others is the primary way to protect your self in a deadly disease.

## Social Distancing

The workout of social distancing is suggested at some stage in pandemics. If you need to be out and round people, it is great to stay as a minimum 6 ft from them. This guarantees you obtained't are available touch with their germs spread via droplets. If aerosol transmitted ailments are gift, it's miles endorsed to live as masses as 30 feet away. Avoid sharing commonplace regions and avoid areas using community air go with the drift systems like place of business homes.

Quarantine

Typically, quarantines are belief of to isolate inflamed human beings, or suspected instances of infection, from the healthful populace. This isolation limits the form of humans the infectious infection can unfold to. When the unfold of a illness reaches the element in which it is uncontrollable through quarantining the unwell, it's miles often crucial to isolate each person in the on the spot populace. This "shotgun" method is generally a final-ditch attempt and reduce the spread of contamination to viable numbers.

Both social distancing and quarantines are presupposed to starve the disease out thru using getting rid of their deliver of replica that is new uninfected people.

Hygiene

Hygiene for every humans and surfaces is essential to reduce the unfold of infectious sickness. When contact can't be avoided, it is important to scrub surfaces that humans can come into touch with to take away any infectious particles. To growth the effectiveness, and compensate for any lapse, washing the frame elements that usually come into contact with probably contaminated surfaces is likewise useful.

Dangerous Confusion

Some agencies have considered one in every of a kind strategies to speak risks and protection precautions. This lack of synchronization can be unstable for the overall public because of the truth it could create a fake understanding of precautions vital to defend a population from infectious illness.

If one agency claims the virus is droplet however moreover may be inhaled if you're indoors 6 feet, some businesses may additionally keep in mind droplet NOT to be an inhalation chance. Inhalation danger designations are every so often reserved exceptional for aerosols. This is a loophole a few companies can use to "actually" tell populations they don't want masks for safety. You will understand even as this is going on because of the reality masks may be mandated for healthcare personnel to shield THEM from the inhalation transmission hazard3.

As noted, inhalation of droplets is idea to be from internal 6 feet, however there have been stated instances of people turning into sick in quarantines wherein they'll handiest have in all likelihood shared one element, air float. That has been stated in each condo houses and cruise ships. When the transmissibility appears so excessive, it'll beg the question, "Why now not advise mask as a precaution?"

Nearly all scientific researchers and primary responders take a function of maximum protecting levels besides a risk is diagnosed to require a awesome deal much much less protection. This is the region you need to take too.

THINK.

Increased Risk Factors

Just as with every infectious illness, there are various not unusual danger factors that increase your probability of becoming inflamed. Traveling through areas in which people have mentioned to be inflamed, being round quite a few people, and already stricken by a sickness or having a compromised immune machine are all factors that growth your danger of being inflamed. If one in a million are inflamed with a pandemic (most effective a random range as an example), then your chance of stepping into touch with an inflamed man or woman starts offevolved at 1 in one million and is going up with every new touch. This is a listing of a number of the elements that boom your risk;

- Travel

- Jobs that positioned you in touch with a immoderate quantity of human beings

- Public Transportation

- Medical Professionals and People Who Have Contact with Sick People

- High populated regions and areas with many site visitors

- Public Events

- Tourist Destinations

- Weekend Immune Systems

- Diseases

- Age

- Poor hygiene habits

- Poor food regimen

- Genetics (likely)

It is a steady to anticipate that the previously mentioned hazard elements are all relevant to any present day-day-day pandemic.

How Do Risk Factors Affect You?

The remarkable manner I actually have positioned to place it is to think about a each day lottery. In this lottery even though, you don't win money, you win a illness. I call it the Wu Han Lottery.

Your chances are 1 in 1,000,000 (those aren't your real opportunities however I'm the usage of this big variety for instance). Now, you're a human and this is your one lottery rate tag. Each additional threat detail you have got is some extra lottery tickets. So, you figure in an administrative center building, you are taking public transportation, you're older, and also you attend one social occasion or visit a public place as soon as each week (celebration, restaurant, grocery store, church, and so on). Now you've got a handful of lottery tickets.

The trick to this lottery is that every person you come back into contact with stocks their lottery tickets with you and you proportion your tickets with them. If you are cautious and brilliant have 20 tickets, but your coworker has 200 tickets, now you each have 220 tickets. If you parent in an place of job complete of heavy rate tag holders, you could have tens of lots of tickets via the prevent of the day. Then you're taking your tickets home and the entire circle of relatives shares its tickets in a unmarried massive pool.

Get the idea?

The real information is the lottery resets every day. You can also reduce the big form of tickets you acquire thru how many threat elements you avoid.

As with any lottery, on this lottery you may have 900,000 tickets and regardless of the truth that no longer agreement an infectious sickness. Conversely, you can have one price ticket and win.

Typical pandemics are quite contagious in case you come into contact with someone who is unwell for any period of time. They unfold with out hassle and similarly so if humans are regularly getting into contact with different people, like in cities. There are severa factors that make it tough to because it must be kingdom how contagious a disorder is:

- Under said because of mild symptoms and signs and symptoms and symptoms

- Under stated due to people toughing it out

- Under recommended because of fear of ramifications


- Misreported due to misdiagnosis


- Not enough sorting out abilities


- Not sufficient hospital beds/ people being grew to emerge as away


- People quarantined and staying in their domestic


The misdiagnosis isn't a moderate on the clinical community. Misdiagnosis is regularly instances smooth to do and doesn't purpose catastrophe very frequently in any respect. If you've visible 50 patients inside the past 5 days and they have all had the flu, and also you display up with flu signs and signs and symptoms, bet what you'll probable be diagnosed with? The flu. They may additionally moreover run a check to affirm, however you'll be encouraged you likely have the flu and given treatment for the flu.

I'd additionally like to say, in case you're now not examined and showed to have a specific infection, then you definitely don't officially have it. Many people can be calling into hospitals complaining of signs and symptoms and signs and symptoms and is probably encouraged to live home in voluntary quarantine with out being tested. Some of them may in the end die at domestic. Do you accept as true with you studied they could be losing take a look at kits on humans who have died? Do you found folks who ought to have died are being counted?

THINK.

Why Data is Important

When some component isn't recommended, or is misreported, the facts used to investigate the spread of similar or associated ilnesses isn't correct. We can pass decrease again and feature a have a look at the information for beyond outbreaks and discern out how contagious they had been, how many people were severely ill, and how many human beings died. We can do this due to the truth we've statistics. Now that the incident has stopped it's far simpler to test out the inflamed areas, ask questions, or maybe easy up a number of the statistics. We can then check excellent figuring out elements and show how severity and contagiousness modified from tradition to life-style or area to region.

The data subjects lots less for the preceding outbreak and more so for the subsequent outbreak. Early on in an event where a state-of-the-art infectious ailment seems, we may moreover perceive a similar or associated contamination. This might in all likelihood permit us to use the records from a previous outbreak and use it as a baseline for the current outbreak. We can then start to make predictions as to the unfold and that would tell us the quantity of essential response.

If the records isn't accurate, we can be at the back of the power curve and no longer respond in time to save you the unfold. It have to virtually propose the difference among 1,000 infections and one million infections.

The information is useful in contemporary times to peer how a virulent disease could be responding to our measures to lessen the unfold, like voluntary quarantine and telling the populace that masks don't art work. If the bargain of the unfold is minimal inside the first few weeks, it is probably because of the truth human beings aren't taking it crucial sufficient. It additionally can be due to the fact the authorities didn't take a look at enough inside the starting and their measures did paintings, however we wouldn't be capable of degree it efficaciously till later.

The facts is important. It is our score card in the fight in competition to an epidemic. There are many innings and every one is its personal achievement or failure tale.

## R0

To apprehend how contagious an infectious illness is you need to understand how the unfold is measured, calculated, and what impacts those calculations.

The R0 (suggested "R naught"), is the degree of methods contagious a illness is. It's a mathematical time period used to outline the reproduction amount. In order for a sickness to spread it has to breed, the R0 is a useful tool in speakme contagiousness4.

The R0 gives you the average range of humans one inflamed person will possibly infect. If you've got were given an R0 of five then each inflamed person will probably infect five. This is a mean and because of this one infected individual can infect zero and some other can infect 10 and the commonplace is probably an R0 of five.

The R0 is useful in predicting how fast an infectious disorder can unfold which offers those tasked to combat the sickness an fantastic idea of how robust the quarantine and social distancing measures need to be. Many times, it's far used misleadingly and may be taken to mean the particular increase fee.

The R0 will become tough to decide if vaccinations are delivered to the equation. The hazard elements stated in the preceding economic catastrophe can also have an effect at the R0 of a metropolis, metropolis, state, and the us. Education and property also have an impact. Access to smooth water, modern-day scientific centers, schooling, running water and cleansing cleaning soap all play a component, even in 2020. Culture can on occasion play are feature however probable not as often.

Politics is in truth playing a function in cutting-edge outbreaks. If one element overplays it, the other difficulty will manifestly underplay it, and no one will remember accurate records even because it comes out. Which technique no individual will realize the fantastic strategies to protect themselves.

The Mortality Numbers Game

If anyone acknowledges there are unreported instances who've an infectious disorder and get better, then you definitely definately truely furthermore want to renowned there are unreported times who have the sickness and die. If they've the disorder and get higher then they don't depend range in opposition to the totals, however the equal may also go for those who've the disorder and die. No?

Because deaths which might be unconfirmed are also disregarded of the totals, I don't recollect each at the same time as thinking about a presently encouraged mortality charge. I expect that might be irresponsible and unethical. Unless I knew a person modified into failing to file showed times, thereby placing their thumb at the scales, I may genuinely take the numbers as they present themselves.

I have a have a look at the statistics that technological information has continuously favored, the totals from closed instances. If a case is open, how do you recognize what the very last effects may be? So in case you study all active and closed instances together, and then try to derive a mortality rate form that, haven't you artificially deflated the mortality charge?

If we test the variety of closed instances and characteristic a examine the possibilities of people who each got higher, or didn't, then we come to the most correct modern mortality price. So, proper here are the numbers once more:

Total Closed Cases = Cured + Deaths giving us Mortality Rate of X%

During a plague it is probably too early to inform what the actual mortality fee might be as there are such loads of factors as a manner to play into the occasion as time went on. I admit this could be a superficial have a test the numbers, however I am showing you this because of the fact the numbers the governments and records media might be placing out, are less close to the entire photo than those might be.

Testing might be the nice way to decide many components of a deadly disease. However, early on it is probably tough to create a test package deal as time might be had to check any new illness. Then the time to manufacture and supply the test kits might probably variety with the aid of availability of producing facilities and any particular substances required.

Even if there had been sufficient check kits, finding out for a ailment might not be as smooth as attempting out for pregnancy. Early on, samples might want to be sent off to notably solid labs for finding out. There are only a few of those labs within the international. These labs are also no longer installation to test tens of hundreds of samples a day.

This way a sickness may be spreading during South Asia, Africa, and the Middle East and nobody may want to understand till it come to be blatantly apparent. At this aspect the arena might in all likelihood already be inside the lower back of the energy curve for locating out and quarantine; quarantine being the best treatment a number of the countries can offer the infected. Because of feasible mask shortages, clinic bed shortages, and terrible medial staffing, quarantine is the pleasant safety most worldwide locations can provide.

Recovery Rate

As to no longer be overly doom and gloom, the other facet of the coin may additionally display us that there may be generally normally a fantastic recuperation price. A healing rate at the better kind of 90% is promising from a pandemic mindset. Unlike other pandemics, in modern instances if you live to tell the tale contamination you received't be referred to as a witch and stoned to demise or burned alive, in order that's a plus.

One ray of moderate is that there were numerous scientific breakthroughs in present day-day instances. You may want to count on to peer opinions of recent sicknesses being handled or even cured with various medicinal pills which have been currently in use and manufacturing.

These ought to variety from a mixture of to be had capsules to experimental ones. We ought to pay attention of medical trials of new pills and if the fulfillment reminiscences have been real, then it might be simplest a count of time in advance than a healing remedy plan is formalized and applied. This could possibly, of course, have an effect on the Recovery Rate in a remarkable way.

Could a latest Infectious Disease be Here to Stay?

From an evolutionary factor of view, a new disease ought to need to mutate itself out of compatibility with people. From a tactical viewpoint we'd must starve it out through quarantine and immunizations.

If it only took some years to mutate and make itself soar into a new species, then theoretically, it want to most effective take a few years to mutate and make itself leap out as properly. Lessons from influenza might tell us in any other case.

The SARS outbreak appears to have "run its route" and pretty a extremely good deal disappeared. The very last mentioned SARS case end up in 2004. The MERS virus has persevered to pop its head up however that appears to be due to the reality camels appear so as to deliver it. In 2019 there had been 212 instances of MERS.

There have been specialists announcing that we also can additionally in no manner be rid of a state-of-the-art infectious illness. It end up presently advocated that a cutting-edge illness can also circle the globe just like the flu does each year5. If this were the case it may have a massive effect on the global population, specifically in lesser developed international places. The commonplace lifestyles expectancy can also in all likelihood be impacted.

## Chapter 5: How Governments Fight A Pandemic

The first component a central authority does to combat an epidemic is to marshal its medical network. Being informed is the finest form of leverage a government can have. It will evaluate the outbreak with present day-day and capability capabilities and then decide on a plan. Adjustments to the plan will take location because the real war is fought but the sources are almost constantly the equal. The techniques and equipment are commonly the identical too.

Finding the Origin

A new illness that might by no means were visible earlier than, may want to revel in an almost magical price of mutation. Many scientists are quick to assert some component can mutated from a bat virus, to a civet virus, after which to a human virus in what might seem like weeks. This is all genuinely guesswork as there isn't enough evidence to signify something apart from feasible similarities in the RNA.

Typically, origins are not common by means of manner of technological understanding until lengthy after the outbreak has run its course. You can't have an epidemic that infects a couple of species at a time so finding precise species of viruses isn't always viable. At nice you may search for noticeably similar viruses and link the two that manner.

Developing a Vaccine

There may be no regarded vaccine for a brand new illness, despite the fact that there could typically be masses of rumors. There can be groups of scientist on foot diligently on this, and that might be actually manageable. No take into account the manner you test the accomplishment of locating a vaccine, be it altruistic, private benefit, fame, or company greed, all of them point within the course of sufficient motivation to be assured no person can be drawing close to it causally. Everyone might be setting their whole weight into locating a vaccine or therapy. I truly endure in mind this.

Developing a Treatment

It is rumored that pharmaceutical agencies take delivery of as right with there is extra profits in developing a remedy than a remedy. This seems reasonable given the large kind of horribly stories we've heard approximately organizations putting monetary benefit over public protection.

There may be a few promising trials taking region for the use of medicine already in existence to assist treat a virulent disease. Every u . S ., and every subset of their clinical groups, is probably attacking the disorder from extraordinary angles. I might acquire as actual with that if a drug, or combination of medication, turn out to be obtainable that would have an effect on affected character survivability, then it's going to probably be placed rapid. It might not be a remedy, however if it may assist survivability in any way, it might be used.

The governments should deliver restrictions on drug researches however the reality that that could be risky. I wager huge gambles may have large rewards. I without a doubt wish there are is probably no hidden and accidental effects.

What is a Public Health Emergency?

In the United States, A public fitness emergency statement is an movement that releases assets meant to cope with an real or functionality public fitness catastrophe. It gives the federal government the ability to call one of a kind businesses into movement and offer investment for emergency efforts that close by authorities budgets may not have the ability to attend to. It moreover gives the federal authorities the energy to name upon the navy to provide help. Public fitness emergencies had been called for smaller localized emergencies affecting a metropolis or america, and big state-substantial failures.

Epidemic vs Pandemic

An Epidemic is whilst a infection spreads thru a huge part of a population over a pretty brief term.

A Pandemic is an endemic that spreads for the duration of a large area like a continent, more than one continents, or around the globe.

A pandemic is largely a plague that is taking place in more than one nations at one time. An instance is probably at the same time as explorers added illness to South America, it changed into first a community epidemic. It changed into localized to the area in which the "explorers" had been conquering. Eventually it have come to be a pandemic and unfold at some stage in the Americas. However, as it turn out to be contained to the Americas it is able to be argued that it become an endemic as it became localized to the Americas. It didn't re-infect Europe, Asia, Australia, or Africa. The Black Death is considered a Pandemic because it unfold within the direction of most of Europe and slightly into Asia and Africa. If it looks like hair splitting that's because it probably is.

This hair splitting is important due to the fact the distinction amongst an epidemic and pandemic is important even as attempting to find assist from one-of-a-kind worldwide places and international organizations.

Also, as the WHO has reminded us, the optics of a virus usually has an effect on investment markets and country wide economies.

What Could Happen in a New Pandemic?

Nobody has a crystal ball. We have technological understanding, we've got history, and we have were given knowledgeable guesses whole of bias and reviews. As I've been writing this e book topics contemporary activities appear to exchange every day.

Everyone has an opinion and there is probably loads of people that look like overly calming humans down. I wouldn't want to take a bet at their motives, however I do inspire you to THINK about why someone is calling you to take into account a positive angle. Even me.

As I've noted formerly, the definition of a Pandemic is an endemic over a big geographic area that is affecting a large proportion of the population.

Would we prevent genuinely short of a international catastrophe or are we able to walk proper through that door. It is probably determined with the useful resource of methods society, you and I, react. The responsiveness of the scientific and the clinical community may also help appreciably.

Like Influenza A New Disease Could be with us Forever

There are some scientists already making statements that a modern infectious ailment might also need to likely be with us all of the time like the flu (See preceding talk). Because a brand new outbreak want to spread so fast and without issue, there wouldn't be an lousy lot optimism amongst some doctors and scientists. Doubts that the world is probably able to contain a virus to a degree in which it'll die off may need to run immoderate. Especially if a present day micro organism or virus also appeared to be hardy sufficient to face as much as warmer climates from early signs.

There can also be reviews that it can be viable to end up infected with the identical contamination extra than as quickly as which can see it soar round to folks that've already had it. This might endorse the cells would possibly mutate in the identical manner the flu does so the frame's antibodies wouldn't prevent reinfection. There may be a couple of separate lines so it can be feasible to get infected separately thru a couple of model.

If we couldn't save you the spread inside the northern hemisphere, and the illness survives the summer season months within the southern hemisphere, then there may be a chance this may spread and evolve. That might make vaccination hard simply as it is hard with the flu. The modern flu vaccines are best approximately forty% effective in step with the CDC net web page. Now forty% is better than not whatever, however the ones aren't suitable betting odds.

If we were to take defensive measures for people in the excessive-chance classes, then it's far feasible to anticipate sending the closing low hazard population again to artwork and a without a doubt regular lifestyles. This could probable assist economies and offer infrastructure guide for those excessive-risk humans living in a few form of quarantine. We might want to create a today's normal till a vaccine or appropriate remedy emerge as acquired.

As a impact, want to it come to be seasonally international just like the flu, there will be a number of preliminary deaths and transfers of wealth. There might be a whole lot of senior assignment openings and a number of out of place expertise and records. I can't in reality fathom the full impact if it were to become a seasonal outbreak.

It might be that there may be exceptional medical treatments that increase the survivability quickly after the initial wave. I don't recognise how powerful they is probably, however I recollect it would extensively lessen the dearth of lifestyles toll. Will there be lasting outcomes? Will there no matter the truth that be a comparable severity requiring a few hospitalization?? There are an entire lot of questions as to how lots of an impact technological know-how should have in this.

## Dealing with a pandemic

A pandemic resolves itself in one in every of methods, each the virus or bacteria dies on its private or we kill it. That's truly about it. There may additionally need to always be a big meteor that solves the problem but then we wouldn't be involved about a bargain after that, so we'll truly maintain targeted on the ones .

## The Disease Dies Off

There are a pair techniques the illness can die off. First, and like many germs, it can be tormented by heat climate. In this case the cells don't remaining prolonged outdoor of the body in warm weather and due to this the R0 is appreciably reduced to a great deal less than 1. This cut charge sees the spread dwindle till it is long lengthy past. If the sickness regarded to be spreading inside the southern hemisphere, which can be currently playing summer season climate, this will not be a truth.

The second way it is able to die off is through mutation. Mutation is what would have made it properly proper with people so it's miles feasible that mutation must make it incompatible with humans. There isn't always any telling how lengthy this could take for the reason that shape of possible mutations important for a ailment to bypass species is unknown. Sadly, this appears to be every different prolonged shot.

## We Kill the Disease

Humans are accurate at finding strategies to kill stuff. We seem to have an first-rate knack for it, in spite of the fact that unintended at times. Given sufficient motivation and sources, people can do masses of harm. The scientific community can be racing for a treatment. The pharmaceutical network will be racing for a therapy. Together, they ought to be quite ambitious fighters of a modern day disease.

No be counted amount which direction the sickness takes, one hit marvel or seasonal traveler, we would desire to in the end have a vaccine that made an impact. Vaccines take some time to make bigger, and they must. We have seen what can seem even as vaccines are rushed thru trials and the consequences were horrifying. There isn't always any gain in having a vaccine to shield you from a sickness that is going to present you maximum cancers or cripple you for lifestyles. To the medical community, I might say, "take the time and get it proper."

We apprehend guidelines should possibly be lifted but there would continually be want for non-public duty a number of the clinical and studies agencies.

In the intervening time there would probably possibly already treatment tablets within the trial ranges. Treatment pills take plenty a good deal less time to check and for that reason take masses much less time to get to the market. Some of those drugs is probably already available on the market. I'm certain there might be errors and accidental results there too. It is the man or woman of the game sadly.

A treatment seems to be more likely than a new disorder loss of existence off, however it could be a close to race. It is a race that people win no matter who locations or indicates (a touch horse making a bet humor from my Grandfather).

What Could Make Things Worse

Panicking is on the top of the list for growing a situation worse. A elegant panic might see the ongoing selling off of stocks, the meals keep shelves staying empty, and possibly a few rioting endeavors in which people pick up the profession of looting for a few days. That constantly makes topics worse. It continues human beings in a fight-or-flight state and that isn't a awesome prolonged-term wondering country of mind.

As the variety of infected climbs our clinical resources and ability might be examined. If we aren't making plans and getting prepared a long manner enough in advance then we are able to typically appear to be seeking to entice up. I may inspire anyone to allow their government to overreact a touch so they'll be prepared to deal with a barely large epidemic than they're hoping for. If it looks as if the system can control it there can also be tons lots much less panic.

Less panic accurate. More panic bad.

If a provider like strength, communications, or water are interrupted it would be a compounding problem. If multiple services are interrupted, it would devolve right right into a poop show fast. Pun meant, I bet. We need our current-day conveniences to offer for our health. We need refrigeration, warm temperature, and a few even need clinical devices to get at the facet of for each day life. We don't salt our meats, make bigger a lawn, or have wooden stoves anymore so the ones are necessities that we are able to't stay with out for extraordinarily extended.

If the deliver chain gets disrupted, then you definitely received't want to worry about save cabinets emptying as it's been ransacked. If there aren't any resupply vehicles, it might empty on its personal. This isn't that massive of an difficulty so long as there's gas and willing drivers besides the pandemic became great lethal. If imports bogged down, or maybe save you, some of the sphere stores is probably empty however that obtained't be too worrisome besides for the stock marketplace. It is the food transport vans that depend maximum within the quick time period. We produce sufficient meals in America to feed ourselves, so our manufacturing functionality isn't a issue.

There is a saying, "The Thin Blue Line," and it speaks to the idea that law enforcement, and their perceived functionality to manipulate justice, are all that stand in the manner between a lawful society and anarchy. There is a lot to that. Hurricane Katrina furnished the location examples of simply how critical that thin blue line is to a society. If they lose their capacity to hold lawlessness to a minimal, then against the law spree should get terrible.

Oddly enough, returning to everyday life ought to make things worse if it's far finished too short. If the sickness continues to be lingering inside the network, there might be a resurgence worse than the preliminary outbreak. This is because of the truth an preliminary cluster includes a affected character 0, the primary character to unfold the disease. A resurgence will possibly have many affected person zeros that unfold the disease, so it then spreads faster.

Likewise, if journey guidelines were lifted, or they weren't put in region quick sufficient, the sickness ought to hop round even faster that may offer dizzying flow infection. When you couldn't trace the sickness to where someone had gotten inflamed with it, it becomes "Community Spreading" and this is at the same time as you're beginning to play entice up.

The lack luster and reactionary response via most governments might be making topics worse. Until the government have turn out to be proactive and regarded to do subjects in a manner that seemed like overreacting, the disease may also want to hold to spread.

To preserve calm and keep away from political outcomes, the authorities would probable probable supply people a faux experience of safety and that could help the illness unfold due to the truth they gained't be on shield. This isn't conspiracy precept. This is out of the playbooks of every unit I supported.

Finally, the pandemic must grow to be very politicized. Politics makes no longer something better. The disorder doesn't care approximately your politics and will hold to spread because of shortsightedness and political dreams. I can also blame each components. Anyone willing to push fear mongering and panic, understanding the opposition birthday celebration will offer a counter message, for political benefit is evil. If that 1/2 america of a will take a dangerously informal technique simply because of the reality you are politically weaponizing the ailment and keep to accomplish that is just EVIL. Anyone at the way to neglect approximately statistics and encourage others to dismiss records, placing them in a dangerously compromised state of affairs, to guard their political candidate is actually STUPID.

What Could Make Things Better

If the world unified and took on an method to protect its citizens over its GDP, we'd see a global change for the higher.

It appears that SARS have come to be killed off with the aid of a mixture of climate and quarantine. Silver lining to Global Warming? (Just kidding.) The final stated instances of SARS have been lab-based totally definitely infections due to carelessness in a Chinese lab, in 2004. This technique the virus lasted from late 2002 till sooner or later in 2004. It best unfold to definitely below eight,000 showed instances so I'm afraid it is able to no longer be apples to apples in as some distance as how contagious a present day illness can be.

Vaccines need to obviously make things higher. So may need to effective treatments that lower the severity of the sickness. I've mentioned those already, so I'll circulate on.

Awareness is high. I can't pound this into your head enough. Staying updated on what is happening with a plague, and for your network location specifically, will be one of the fine defensive measures you could take. If all of us took it critically and lived in a defensive posture concerning the sickness for only a few months, it might contain itself as a substitute short. Any sickness desires dwelling hosts to live alive and if we robbed the disease of that, it might die off. Think about what the government and your enterprise        enterprise        enterprise        are recommending and take it only a step further and you'll in all likelihood be proper at the right tune.

Working from domestic is a exquisite present day device in lowering the unfold of an infectious illness. By running from home you're continuing to make contributions to the economic device via making sure the continuity of your business enterprise. I understand this pleasant relates to a small percentage of people in the modern-day-day-day staff. But if you can clean out an place of job building of ninety% of the personnel you may reduce the opportunities of spreading the illness substantially. Office houses take masses of people and stuff all of them into the equal field, sharing the same heating, ventilation, and cooling (HVAC) device. The HVAC system can spread the germs via partitions and amongst floors. In only a few days one character can infect lots. Those loads then bypass directly to infect others on their way home and in their every day lives. Seems unnecessary inside the event that they can be even remotely as effective running from domestic.

Home shipping of meals might reduce the amount of human beings out and approximately as properly, as compared to consuming out. I apprehend, if a prepare dinner dinner or shipping person is infected, they'll probable infect others. So, warmth, or reheat meals approximately one hundred sixty five and 212 degrees Fahrenheit for 10 mins or more. Use a food thermometer. I have been given a cheap little one like this, Amazon link: Pocket Size Food Thermometer and it does super. You can spend as masses as you need despite the fact that.

The factor is, in case you're ordering meals, or maybe looking for glowing food that has been dealt with, you'll want to elevate the temperature to at least one hundred sixty 5 degrees for 10 mins to cast off the danger from micro organism and viruses. Now the heat may not technically "kill" a virulent disease as it isn't technically "alive," but it will circulate dormant rendering it secure to devour or it will decompose.

The shipping person would probable contaminate the outside of containers so placed on gloves whilst dealing with ordered food. Bring it proper to the counter and start cleaning it. Decontaminate it and get rid of the packaging as it must be. You'll help preserve the eating place organisation alive and enhance morale with a delectable dish.

I do no longer apprehend the precise temperatures to kill viruses and bacteria so please do your very very own studies to verify those numbers.

Lately I've commenced the use of grocery transport services known as Peapod. My referral code gets you 60 days loose delivery and $25 off of your first orders over $seventy five: https://peapod.Extole.Com/s/Jason142 . Instead of walking spherical a shop entire of people and coming head to head with the cashier, or the use of a touch show display utilized by hundreds of others with questionable hygiene, I were given a delivery the alternative day of spherical $200.00 properly without a doubt really worth of groceries and spent an entire 30 seconds near the delivery character. When smart is also clean, it's a bonus. I went from being in near proximity to 15 to two hundred human beings, to simply 1. I furthermore much like the truth that you could't purchase out a whole keep of a few aspect due to the fact their purchasing cart flags you at like 10 or some issue similar. I had been given 10 cans of carrots and it gave me a crimson caution over the "add to cart" button. Seems like a reasonably accountable degree in instances wherein belongings may be scarce.

A phrase of warning, I presently had an order scheduled but needed some gadgets in advance than my shipping. I went looking for and used my bonus card. The organisation tracks all of my purchases thru that bonus card. Shortly as quickly as I arrived domestic, I got an automated message affirming that my delivery have been canceled and the meals have grow to be located once more into my purchasing cart. I am assuming this grow to be intentional and a guard closer to hoarding. While I applaud it, I want they might have compared the 2 carts with my records of meals buy. They would have seen I had a own family of five, and a canine, and purchase meals pretty regularly. Keep that in thoughts at the same time as the use of delivery offerings. Who is aware about how they may track and regulate purchase inside the destiny?

If we, as a society, moved to a version of self-imposed quarantine where we only went out of doors even as essential, then topics should right away start looking up. I mean, you will reduce your opportunities and so could likely anyone else. I'm not saying to in no way flow into out of doors, surely decrease it. If you felt a touch cabin fever, then you may cross for a stroll but sincerely maintain a first rate distance of some yards from others.

If you actually need to be spherical others, you need to vicinity on a mask, some kind of glove, and wraparound sun shades or goggles. This will reduce your possibilities of being infected and decrease your opportunities of spreading it to others if you have it and are unaware. Simple steps like this can in reality retard the unfold of an infectious illness. Definitely skip the social activities and things like change indicates and stay shows.

Then there's constantly the Hand of God, miracle, success, karma, or some thing you be given as real with in. Devine intervention has helped us people out more than as fast as whilst handling global variety. Pray, moderate a candle, mild some incense, put on your pajamas interior out, or some thing it's far you do for some supernatural need.

Levels of Emergency

In the early days there could probable look like no real emergency. The majority of the warnings we might be getting can be to easy your arms and get a flu shot. Even with all people being sent home and businesses final their doorways, humans will be wandering round like they're on a spring excursion.

But all of us might be looking the numbers I guess.

I will destroy down a possible situation into 3 levels of emergency so we can wrap our heads spherical them. This is vital because of the fact if we're capable of recognize tiers and associate them with possible influences on our lives, we are able to form of in shape those to our protecting or protecting measures. That being stated, I will try and in shape up defensive measures into 3 levels as nicely.

Could be Nothing

A new disease might be not some aspect for the USA. There is a danger that a halt of excursion into the united states from humans originating in global locations with big infected populations, mixed with amazing worldwide places' extreme quarantines, may also additionally need to have contained this out of doors of the us with the aid of the usage of using higher than 95%.

We realise most global locations have admitted they couldn't pick out each case and they would be underreporting the numbers due to the ones boundaries. Of course, we're assuming actually accurate and sincere reporting from many countries that have a information otherwise. Even if there have been a few intentional lies about the numbers, I don't assume they might be that massive with out a leak of records coming from positive organizations.

It is possible that the usage of social distancing and focused quarantines in reality minimizes the spread of a future pandemic which then need to allow the government and clinical community good enough time to prepare for a massive inflow of illnesses. If this happened humans ought to likely be capable of cross returned to art work rapid and absolutely everyone ought to call it a hoax and waste of time.

When a plague is stopped early on, critics come out of the woodwork to speak approximately scare strategies and overreactions. When they don't consist of a virus early on, humans are brief in charge inaction. Sadly, it's far a no-win state of affairs for maximum folks who deal with protective our united states from mass casualty incidents.

How bad it might get is primarily based upon more on how people react and masses an awful lot less on how the authorities reacts.

Levels of Disaster

So, levels of disaster... inside the context of a worldwide pandemic, we'll have a take a look at three feasible ranges:

- Manageable Spread of the Disease

- Struggle to Contain the Disease

- All Out War on the Disease

Relax a Bit

I'm no longer looking to promote you a rate price tag to mad town. An all-out struggle on a sickness isn't possibly to be continually just like the Netflix specific you observed it's miles. But that diploma of disaster is probably drastic and in reality hard for the common unprepared character. It can also probably regulate their incredible of life and way of lifestyles for a very long time. It is the least possibly scenario, but I wouldn't pull it honestly off the table. If it were to hit you in which you stay, find it irresistible traditionally hits a few smaller global places, buckle up!

## Manageable Spread

Keeping the shape of inflamed of a state-of-the-art infectious disorder to below 3 million humans, a great deal less than 10% of the us populace, should statistically be "possible" in a math sense but no longer in a sensible revel in. If the fee of hospitalization have been to be round 20% it can be devastating.

Let's say because we are America and we're the wonderful at the whole thing (I realize, conceited), we keep it all of the way right down to 10% hospitalization. If so, at 3 million infected we might want three hundred,000 more medical institution beds and docs, nurses, advanced scientific gadget, and factors to help them. We absolutely don't have that and it isn't likely we should get it mobilized that speedy.

If the politicians and the media need to maintain absolutely everyone calm, I think 100,000 and under might be the manageable variety. I anticipate that the United States clinical infrastructure can contend with 10,000 new severely unwell sufferers but possibly no more than that. You want to hold in mind, the ones aren't car coincidence sufferers that may be disregarded in the "open", there are specially contagious people who want to have specific medical quarantine. A wave of 10,000 significantly ill over a few months length, on top of the identical vintage case load of humans rotating through the medical institution, might probable possibly push our assets and innovation to the max.

So my possible spread, or Level three range, is 100,000 infected within the US. I'm now not assured that america should check that many people inside the early infection length. I'm additionally now not exquisite if the government ought to admit to the ones form of numbers early on. It may be in the governments extremely good interest to document one component and advocate every different to the clinical community as "precautionary."

We can slow that down by means of people taking private duty and changing a few behavior. How likely is that? If everybody become selling out of hand sanitizer and facemasks however no character modified into the use of them, then you could take an easy bet? You have to typically appearance to see a change in the amount of people washing their hands in public restrooms maybe?

Struggle To Contain

If it the spread took off in an initial surge like we've visible in preceding pandemics, then brief and drastic measures ought to have to reveal up rapid. I can see a city or falling beneath a quarantine for a few weeks, or months. I'm speaking a metropolis like Atlanta or Baltimore period. Big enough to be a vast logistical hurdle however now not a whole lot past the 5 hundred,000 populace mark.

I apprehend we've appeared to jump from sobering to surreal but as quickly as we get beyond one hundred,000 times there may be probably going to be panic. Even if the numbers are purposely being below mentioned in an try and hold the population calm, every body will start hearing and in my view seeing the effect of the illness.

America could have to pull collectively and aid those cities with donations of each type, and the authorities would possibly need to find out a manner to help the agencies get better financially. Just a few weeks at the proper time of three hundred and sixty five days can truely placed a financial dent in a few bottom traces. This may in reality have a financial impact to excursion, and tourism and they might request billions of dollars in bailouts.

Again, we're looking at 4 to eight weeks perhaps. It might also possibly be voluntary. It may want to begin thru having all non-important employees voluntarily work from home if viable. Essential employees would be asked to take precautionary measures. There may be a small percentage of the populace in which project or fear can also overtake them and they could refuse to move again to art work or outright forestall. Some human beings can be legally required to paintings and threatened with criminal movement by means of the usage of the authorities for refusing.

This Level 2 is a slippery slope. As bizarre because it sounds, people should acquire and start demonstrating and I bear in mind small wallet of rioting will take vicinity after a few weeks. Many ought to need the government to take extra drastic measures. Many will want the government to move away them by myself. The conspiracy theories will start to come to be extra mainstream and might also be discussed to your favorite communicate show.

Level 2 will seem rapid, and it gained't likely last extended. This level is much less approximately the variety inflamed and further about the type of human beings forced to exchange their cushty each day lives through stress and for the way lengthy. It may be a slippery slope for the authorities to tread and it received't take masses of a push to slide into an all-out warfare with the ailment.

All Out War

If we begin seeing numbers honestly established over one hundred,000 then we'd in all likelihood see a central authority quarantine enforced in numerous components of america. This is what I call Level 1.

In the army we used to art work a subject scale in which 1 become the top priority in order that's surely what I'm used to.

I understand, it seems draconian however what a few global locations have completed with excessive quarantines within the past is right out of the emergency playbooks of many military devices that specialize in bioweapon and pandemic reaction. It has the appearance and experience of draconian because of the popularity of some international locations have however nearly speaking it become proper at the coins.

The complete communist like quarantine might be devastating for our economic gadget, similar to I might have assumed this to be devastating for others. Others can also ramp up their production centers early in advance than the quarantine has completely worked and could in all likelihood be loaning money to global locations spherical the arena. They will be set to attain pretty the windfall from the pandemic they will have commenced out.

It would likely sound bloodless to recognition at the coins more than the dying toll but if a rustic takes a large monetary hit to the GDP and tax coffers, easy public offerings need to prevent going for walks. I'm hoping the navy contingency may plan to take over public offerings and utilities to offer continuity, however that wouldn't be a guarantee. All authorities agencies struggle with the "tribal understanding" problem and there can be some interruptions in offerings.

The extra disruption to our manner of lifestyles and normalcy bias, the more the panic and outrage. The greater the panic and outrage, the more the instability in the conduct of the population. Start considering how people behaved inside the route of the Hurricane Katrina occasion.

It can also bankrupt a few agencies to the factor that utilities could be impacted besides the government got here in with stimulus coins. A national 3- or 4-week quarantine is probably tough to drag off. I don't assume all non-crucial personnel might look at it. I anticipate there might be rippling nearby quarantines that is probably like aftershocks. The localized outbreaks may want to possibly preserve going on.

It might be a massive number, and it would be months till we were given matters under control. I don't expect maximum humans may additionally need to move for a month or greater below a quarantine without essential hardships. I suppose humans might lose jobs, clinical medical insurance, financial financial savings and retirements, and perhaps even homes without government intervention.

I hate to sound like a awful prepper movie however all my time in and across the first responder community in reality does thing to the ones troubles being a probable situation if a plague isn't controlled. This situation ought to last up to 6 months or longer relying on how tough the sickness is to embody.

I'm going to stop this thing right proper right here because it usually appears to spiral into despair and some dystopian Mad Max movie. I don't think so one may be the case, so I received't bypass in addition.


This is NOT the Apocalypse

I need to make a easy statement right here for all and sundry who may probable have become labored up analyzing the last few sections: This is possibly no longer doomsday and likely wouldn't be the apocalypse. We may likely undergo a pretty difficult patch and that could likely closing some months or possibly a 12 months. We will see some semblance of regular again afterwards.

World War 1 killed 30 million people. World War 2 killed 80 5 million human beings. The Black Death killed 2 hundred million human beings. Recently, the Spanish Flu killed amongst 30 and a hundred million humans. While those sports activities frighten and scar the population that witnesses them, life is going on. Our records books are full of billions of struggle and plague deaths.

It is probably terrible to stay even though however we, due to the fact the human race, ought to stay through it. You, in case you're studying this ebook, are even much more likely to stay via it due to the reality you're being proactive in your technique.

# Chapter 6: How To Protect Yourself In A Pandemic

If you aren't acquainted with Hazardous Materials or Weapons of Mass Destruction a number of this could sound lots less sane. I encourage you to do a number of homework for your personal.

Now, I'm now not telling you that you shouldn't pass absolutely doomsday prepper. If you sense that's what you want to do, and you've got got the way to do it, then have at it. The assured manner to not be in any risk from a pandemic in any manner is to no longer be round for it. The majority of us don't have the high-priced.

The future may also need to herald improvements from more than one instructions that boom our survivability. You honestly in no way recognize.

The maximum important thing to recollect is DON'T PANIC.

## Links

In the subsequent pages I can be linking to examples and assets. In the later pages I can be going over objects I in fact have personal tales with or the greater moderen fashions of some aspect I even have had experience with. I virtually don't need to tell without a doubt every person to accumulate something I actually have in no manner used or visible in use. So, I will percentage my revel in. There may be better stuff available, and time allowing, I inspire you to do your homework before making any choices.

In almost all instances I am recommending a few element I actually have enjoy with. Most of it I already very very own. When it doesn't rely, like Charcoal grills as an instance, I will do my first rate to reference some thing with well reviews, but I might not hyperlink to the precise grill I sincerely have or have had enjoy with. If it had been mask or handheld atmospheric attempting out gadget, then I could possibly pleasant link to objects I knew well and had enjoy with.

If I come upon a few trouble that I haven't had private enjoy with however feel the need to advise looking into it as an preference, I promise I've researched the object. I don't purchase matters that my existence might possibly rely upon earlier than learning them thru literature and asking humans with firsthand data.

While I don't assume everybody enjoys overpaying, I do preserve in mind you want to pay what you watched your lifestyles is really worth for a few things. I supply an example of creating a mobile phone cleaning bundle deal later in this bankruptcy and endorse locating a manner to preserve it. I thing out the use of a ziplock bag if you can't locate a few thing else. If you are wondering you're going to shop for the cheapest, dollar shop good deal, zip remaining baggage you could locate, don't hassle. Don't hassle purchasing for some component. Save that cash on your funeral prices and next of members of the family.

I'm not bashing parents which are frugal or thrifty. I suppose it is a exquisite trait to have. But at the same time as dealing with certain devices, you want to get a minimum stage of awesome to be effective. If you want to buy bargain bleach, reduce rate bathroom paper, cut fee gas, and so forth, exceptional. When it consists of things which is probably protecting you and others from the unfold of an infectious illness, purchase the critical tremendous to do the approach proper. Cut coupons and keep round however buy the crucial excellent.

We need to furthermore apprehend that some human beings might be taking benefit of a disaster as a cash-making possibility. This is terrible and I wish none of you will be doing this. This is a disgusting skip. If the least bit feasible, do not offer them your coins or barter with them. It can be important, I recognize that. If someone ran out and cornered the market on a resource and is growing the costs due to the truth they helped make the useful resource scarce, it is probably the only activity in town after which you have not any desire. Do what you revel in you need to do but hold the ones people accountable later.

Look at the entirety within the context supplied and THINK.

Current Steps

I enjoy silly writing some of the ones steps I'm recommending however the fact is, I without a doubt don't see many human beings training wonderful hygiene these days. I choice this is most effective a evaluation for max of you and you're already doing these items. If not, the day gone by modified into the time to start doing them in case you get my flow.

The first actions you can take are likely the quality to put into impact. I say that wondering from a perspective of the manner plausible they may be for the not unusual individual.

Risk Mitigation Habits

Think of Risk Mitigation Habits as Personal Protection Habits which might be supposed that will help you keep away from touch with germs. Your fine way to avoid touch is to stay in a bubble. That isn't continuously practical for max people. Besides, wherein do you go to the bathroom in case you live in a bubble? If you can't live in a bubble, you then definately simply must do your wonderful to avoid touch.

These practices, that you can change into conduct, will considerably lessen your danger of coming into contact with a extraordinarily contagious infectious illness.

Stop touching unique humans

This could in all likelihood appear apparent, but it'll take workout to alternate conduct so I'm bringing up it right right here. Stop shaking people's hands and hugging them. Some cultures kiss when they excellent and say good-bye. That's all amazing however these gadgets will useful useful resource the disorder in spreading to new human beings. So, within the course of an endemic, take a brake and greet every special from a distance. You can improve a hand to greet like the vintage Native American stereotype or bow from a distance similar to the antique college Japanese. Do some thing you need, genuinely prevent touching each one-of-a-type.

Wash your arms

The next most effective problem you could start doing is washing your arms... often6. Please don't count on you understand the way to easy your fingers. Pride comes in advance than the fall.

Hospitals in reality have education on hand washing. Google right handwashing or appearance it up on YouTube. Make sure that it's miles instructional and now not really theorizing why handwashing is right. You want to apprehend a manner to clean them. The UCLA Heath YouTube channel has a outstanding rationalization right here: https://www.Youtube.Com/watch?V=4E7UkDln vZA.

Wash your palms after doing these items:

How frequently have to you wash your arms? A desired rule is probably, if you can't maintain in thoughts the last time you washed your hands, it might be time to easy your hands. You will cast off any virus AND micro organism which can be on your palms. You don't want to fight the virus best to get a bacterial contamination.

Other than that, right here are a few occasions whilst you want to be which include handwashing on your current-day operating system (SOP):

Before, throughout, and after handling food: You don't want to contaminate the food all up earlier than you and your family devour it. Some meals also can have been infected with germs. Some food also can moreover have bacteria that dies off in cooking however is positioned in uncooked meats and you don't want to unfold that to uncooked food. So wash in advance than touching the meals. Wash the food. Wash arms even as going to and fro many of the meals types and wash up whilst you're completed.

Before eating meals: You don't need to put infection onto the cheeseburger (or kale chip) you're about to shove to your mouth. You moreover want to hold in mind coping with straws and similar smaller activities. Even putting a bit of sweet or cough drop to your mouth is probably a way of get proper of access to into your gadget an infectious contamination takes benefit of. The despite the fact that proper proper right here is you don't need to contaminate a few thing you're installing your mouth.

Before and after annoying for a person at home who is sick: This ought to be obvious however for masses it isn't. If someone has an infectious sickness then they will be breathing it into the air, they'll be expelling it of their sweat, they're throwing it up, and they're pooping it out. Treat a few issue that comes out in their frame as infected. If you're coming into contact with infected surfaces, placed on rubber or latex gloves and then wash up after.

Before and after treating a lessen or wound: We wash in advance than touching a wound, at the same time as succesful and time permitting, because we don't need to area any bacteria or virus into the wound. They're already bleeding, we don't need to make their existence worse. If you can't wash your hands, then you definitely really need to use rubber gloves if to be had. Hand sanitizer as a closing motel. I wouldn't permit the absence of any of these save you you from performing lifesaving medical care, but. Not many viruses are within the blood, however we wash our fingers after besides due to the fact HIV and Hepatitis B & C are real, and we don't need to go back into touch with those either7.

After being bodily placed in a rest room: A lot of humans will provide you with a warning to clean up after using the restroom and this is right, you should. But absolutely being in a lavatory has the capability to infect you8. Forget the reality that humans are coughing and sneezing in bathrooms. Forget that human beings are touching all of these surfaces. It is the toilet I need you to be considering. Even if you don't contact the rest room, the toilet can contaminate you. Toilets can throw microscopic water droplets, much like the ones created sneezing, coughing, and respiration, severa toes away. Here is a YouTube video that comically addresses the subject at the equal time as even though making the component: https://www.Youtube.Com/watch?V=EG_PnRC Le9A.

Public bathrooms have a touch extra stress to prevent clogging, so that they've the capability to throw these droplets in addition. Aside from grossing you out, I'm pointing this out to because of the truth some infectious diseases are fecal-oral transmittable. I recognize, yuck, however to procure to understand this. So whenever you're in a restroom, wash up, and don't live for to any quantity further than you need to. Don't loaf around were given the selfie. You can also want to rinse with an antiseptic as well.

After touching a little one or some thing belonging to a toddler: Babies require diaper converting and often spew fluids of 1 kind or some other from all of the holes in their frame. Any potty-informed little one is probably lacking within the hygiene abilities to well wash up. And there is additionally the opportunity that those small creatures have touched their poop. Kids are so icky! I even have 4 kids and a grandkid, so I revel in certified as a subject rely professional in this difficulty.

If they're more youthful, then you definately definately need to in all likelihood wash them each time you're near them after which wash yourself. At least wash their palms and face. If the usage of wipes, cope with the decontamination in their pores and pores and pores and skin surfaces similar to handwashing as a long way as duration and thoroughness. Be extra cautious across the eyes.

After touching an animal or something belonging to an animal: Animals are a bit higher than kids but now not a bargain. Animals can deliver sickness; however it is unknown if animals can supply all sicknesses. Wash up after dealing with their meals and waste. If you puppy them then hold it in thoughts not to touch your face till you wash your arms.

There end up a record that a canine in Hong Kong had lines of an endemic but it wasn't obvious if the virus emerge as without a doubt hitching a journey or if the animal became an actual issuer.

After blowing your nose, coughing, sneezing, or yawning: Any time your hand is going close to your mouth you are putting germs on it. You received't understand when you have an infectious illness till after you start showing symptoms and symptoms so you'll be spreading it. We need to be aware of our very very own actions and take proper care. If everybody were to be accountable for their very personal actions, germs wouldn't unfold as an extended manner. Always try to entice the release of blowing your nostril, coughing, sneezing, or yawning in a disposable serviette and then dispose of it within the trash. Then flow wash your hands.

Yes, yawning discharges droplets too.

After touching rubbish: If we're throwing viable contaminants inside the garbage can then touching stated rubbish can then it opens you as an awful lot as touch with the illness. If you live with different people, if special human beings have get right of access to to the trashcan, or if there is even the slightest risk you can have positioned a tissue, used face mask, used gloves and so on. Into the trash can, deal with it as probable inflamed fabric. Also, bacteria and one in every of a kind unsightly subjects are placed in trash cans, so it's far truly an wonderful exercising in cutting-edge. Wash your hands whenever deal with rubbish.

Any specific time you discovered you've in all likelihood come into touch with inflamed surfaces: Don't genuinely wash your fingers underneath the above occasions, wash them wherever you positioned it's far a wonderful concept. Don't wash them till they bleed. You're in reality searching for to expand appropriate hygiene conduct.

THINK.

Antibacterial soap and hand sanitizers are not the solution. I'm now not denouncing them. I trust that human beings placed too much bear in mind in them, just like I used to.

Hand Sanitizer

Hand sanitizer is proper for whilst you don't have proper now access to cleaning cleansing soap and water30. If you revel in the want to use hand sanitizer then after you use it, you need to be seeking out an area to scrub your fingers. Handwashing and hand sanitizer art work otherwise with handwashing being the simplest. It is straightforward to expect hand sanitizer can be "suitable enough" but it isn't. It moreover doesn't smash the whole lot. It stays pretty effective, so we don't disregard it or rule it out.

The trouble is that the alcohol wants to be in every corner and cranny that the virus or micro organism can also need to possibly be in. Most humans don't take the time to rub the gel into the ones areas. The gel moreover wants to preserve the alcohol at the pores and skin prolonged sufficient for the alcohol ruin the infection. This calls for a slightly large dose to be accomplished than human beings typically use.

Again, not vain, but simply no longer a alternative for handwashing.

Antibacterial Soap

Handwashing works as it bonds to debris, lets in loosen them from the pores and pores and skin, and then incorporates them away. Because cleansing soap itself doesn't rinse off the pores and pores and skin resultseasily, you spend time rubbing it off your pores and pores and skin and that greater time allows the cleansing soap to seize greater debris to be over excited.

Antibacterial cleaning soap attempts to kill micro organism throughout this technique in order that if any are left on the pores and pores and skin, it will try to kill the final floor infection as well10. While that may be a extremely good idea, there isn't masses of evidence that this truely works. As continuously, the "specific stuff" was probably risky to human beings so it come to be banned with the aid of the FDA.

There was a mandate with the aid of the FDA that agencies qualify the antibacterial declare earlier than a producer ought to sell it. So, there want to be a few usefulness while protecting in opposition to micro organism.

Here is the thing that most people overlook approximately, we can be stopping a virulent disease-based pandemic, no longer a bacterial infection. It is super that we're conscious and of path we don't need to capture a bacterial infection even as shielding in the route of a hastily spreading virus, however we want to THINK. Don't be lulled right into a false experience of safety because of the fact you're using antibacterial cleaning soap. Don't buy up the whole lot genuinely as it says "antibacterial." Again, antibacterial cleaning soap kills micro organism, no longer viruses.

The nuclear bomb of soaps

Hibiclens is an antimicrobial cleansing soap that has been utilized in hospitals for years. It is used for cleaning gadgets and for sterilizing the scientific personnel in addition to sufferers. It uses chlorhexidine gluconate (CHG) which basically breaks down cell walls in viruses and micro organism. While this cleaning cleaning soap washes away like others, the lively additives are left in the returned of, adhering to the pores and pores and pores and skin, running for as an entire lot as 24 hours. This permits the CHG to commonly degrade virus and bacteria cells. It is listed at the World Health Organization's List of Essential Medicines. Hibiclens Antimicrobial Skin Liquid Soap, Amazon hyperlink: https://amzn.To/391AMIW

Moisturize to save you cracks and bleeding

Use a super lotion or moisturizer because you'll be washing your hands greater often. Dry pores and pores and pores and skin can crack and you then definately get those little splits in the pores and pores and pores and skin through the use of your fingertips or your hands could be difficult and bleed without problem. It is a minor nightmare to live with the ones problems and also you don't want to be bleeding everywhere in the region. I apprehend the ones are excessive examples, however it's far a likely one if you're washing up 20 or 30 instances a day and no longer giving your hand any moisture back.

I suffer from dry palms that get splits on the fingertip and feature struggled with it for years. No, it is not a sign of something else. I get bloodwork completed every six months and do yearly physicals. I absorb loads of fluids and people fluids want to go back once more out ultimately. This manner I'm washing my hands frequently. I've tried all forms of creams, however my daughter introduced me to O'Keeffe's Working Hands Hand Cream. It has worked for me, in my state of affairs, very well. They're no longer a sponsor, it's miles just genuinely right lotion that has solved this handwashing associated hassle for me. Here is an Amazon hyperlink: O'Keeffe's Working Hands Hand Cream. If you have already got a pass-to moisturizer that works then stay with that.

Clean your phone

Your cellular telephone is nasty. Wash your cellphone. Not simplest do your palms continuously contact your mobile phone however you supply it anywhere with you, together with the relaxation room. We in reality went over lavatories. If you remember it, washing your palms however no longer washing your phones is type of vain. You're definitely putting the contamination right decrease again onto your hand.

You should make a cellphone washing bundle for every of your bathrooms and one or two for excursion. It is quite smooth: you spray a piece isopropyl alcohol on a display screen material and wipe it throughout for some seconds. It isn't complicated however in particular critical.

Use little spray bottles to hold your cleaning solution of isopropyl alcohol. Any one-of-a-kind cleaner may additionally damage the cellphone show. Don't spray it on the cellphone due to the reality you don't need the alcohol entering into the mobile telephone even though the microphone, speaker, or data ports. Spray the solution at the rag and wipe the telephone in some unspecified time in the future of. Wash your fingers after cleaning the cellular phone. Amazon hyperlinks to three clean products below:

Spray Bottle

Isopropyl alcohol

Screen Cleaning Cloth

Anything plenty less than 70% alcohol gained't kill a plague or bacteria. It additionally needs to have a mixture of purified water in it to paintings. I'm now not getting into the technicalities of it, sincerely Google it if you want to realise more. The alcohol works better than cleaners in the way that it kills the germs and it additionally evaporates so it gained't possibly harm the cellular telephone. Again, spray the fabric and wipe, don't spray the phone.

I don't anticipate it's miles critical to throw the cloths away whenever, however I might trade them out every few days, or every day if you're leaving your house regularly. Don't wash the cloths as some bacteria and virus can live on the wash. Just purchase new ones, they're cheap. If you are washing your smartphone frequently then perhaps a new cloth a day. You don't want to have a large germ fabric to your pocket. The alcohol will kill it however eventually the rag might be saturated with gunk. Bacteria and viruses can disguise from the alcohol in that gunk. I would moreover discover a case or a few issue to area at the least the cloths in so that you're protective them from dust and amazing contaminants. If all else fails, my pass-to is a sturdy ziplock bag.

My mother gave me a UV smartphone sanitizer a few years in the past. I used it a few times and I wager it worked. Technically, the UV need to kill the virus and micro organism if it's far robust enough UV-C slight. The stores say it does work and it probable does do the job. I suppose I is probably antique college and just like the easy enjoy of cleaning it myself. But there is no damage in the use of it, and in case you're lazy, this is probably the outstanding bet. Amazon link: UV Bed Phone Sanitizer. It is better than not cleaning your phone in any respect. If you received't do a high-quality interest of cleansing your cellular phone with the cloths, then my advice is get it.

One manner to lessen the need to sanitize your cellular cellphone is to stay off of it and don't convey it into the rest room. I recognize that frightens most of the populace so surely make your cleaning kits and stash them strategically spherical your own home and work at the equal time as finding a way to hold a package with you. If it's time to scrub your fingers, then it's likely time to easy your cellphone.

The 6 Feet Rule

Early on, you won't realise is an infectious sickness is aerosol and droplet spreading. I endorse that in case you're going to an area in which other people are then put on a masks, wraparound solar sun shades/ goggles, and probably gloves. If a person is coughing or sneezing, they'll be spreading the disease out faster and similarly. Move far from them. If they cough or sneeze on you, don't panic, without a doubt waft away and wash up as fast as you can.

When someone coughs or sneezes, they will be able to unfold their germs up to six ft away. That is a six-foot circle of viable contamination they devise. Don't be mad at them, this is natural. Being filled like sardines in a metro-rail is unnatural. So, if you don't stroll spherical with a surgical masks and someone is interior six ft of you and they're coughing and sneezing, you then simply may want to possibly want to cover your face thru some way. Watch in that you are touching and assume the entirety you contact close to them is infected. Move a stable distance away as soon as you could pretty do so (don't bounce from the transferring teach). When you get a secure distance away, use some hand sanitizer at the manner to discover someplace to wash up.

After being coughed on, address your hat, hair, shirt, pants, skirt, purse, footwear, and anything else on you as in all likelihood infected and wash them as you normally may also want to. Adding some shade stay bleach is likely vital to try to kill the virus and bacteria debris. You can wipe nonporous (smooth surfaces) topics down with the same alcohol you operate to easy your cellphone. It might damage the apparel over time, but it is better than the being infected.

How to be consistent but no longer appearance loopy

It is unhappy that early on in a plague wearing a masks and goggles to protect your self from a virulent disease this is spreading around the arena quicker than the flu makes you look crazy. Aside from the viable incorrect records at the TV and net, wearing a mask and goggles and keeping social distancing is the most essential difficulty you can do to shield yourself and your family from a pandemic. Period. With that stated, if you truely can't supply your self to position on a masks, goggles, and gloves, proper right here is my superb advice to provide you some feasible safety.

Most people don't want to "appearance crazy" and walk spherical in masks and bio-fits however we additionally would like a bit protection, I get it. This isn't too hard to get a few protection. Carrying hand sanitizer doesn't look loopy truely so isn't a huge deal. You won't need to put on a bio-healthful, however you can cover up with lengthy pants and lengthy sleeves. If germs get to your pores and pores and skin, there can be commonly the threat that you contact that location and then touch your face. If you cover up, the virus or micro organism might be trapped in your apparel for some hours/ days, however it is probably more secure.

The purpose you could't decontaminate garb one of a kind that washing it in a device is because the virus and bacteria droplets gets trapped inside the among the fibers of the clothing. However, this will additionally make it greater difficult to pick up whilst you contact the cloth. I'm no longer suggesting you do this but I'm maintaining the included body may also entice the germs and preserve it away from your pores and pores and skin to some extent. I may assume that is probably a chunk better. There isn't always any actual study of this so don't bet your lifestyles on it. The not unusual sense is there, and it is likely higher than uncovered pores and skin. Because illnesses commonly circulate in the iciness, protective up in cold climate won't make you appearance loopy.

Slick garb like processed leather-based-based and plastics commonplace in apparel and rainwear won't lure germ particles and droplets. It might also make it lots less tough to pass alongside. Maybe rethink the bright leather trench coat or rain suit except you are willing to wipe it down with a material dampened with alcohol every so often. FYI, a rain wholesome makes an extraordinary improvised protective healthy with a few changes. These items are much less difficult to decontaminate just so they might be precisely what you want to put on.

## Chapter 7: Mitigate Risk Factors

In the section on Risk Factors I go over distinctive issues that growth your hazard of catching an infectious sickness. You must attempt to reduce your hazard. Some subjects are going to be much less complicated to do than others. If you forestall using public transportation or adventure sharing, then your excursion fees might probable pass up (on the aspect of stress ranges). Figure out what you could do after which get on it.

Doorknobs

Doorknobs are definitely worse than bathrooms. Just don't forget it. I'll wait.

Now that you're grossed out, plan to disinfect your doorknobs quite frequently. As for public doorknobs, carrying a small bundle deal of napkins or tissues is incredible for even as you're forced to the touch doorknobs. There isn't an entire lot more to say approximately it.

Treat the napkins and tissues as infected. Fold inward from the outside and eliminate them right away.

If you need to use a manual push shape of door, attempt to use your elbow if you can, to hold on the napkins and tissues. Remember your garb might be infected and act effectively.

Yuck.

Permanent and Temporary

You have to consider making a number of these behavior permanent. Handwashing want to be on the pinnacle of that listing. However, I don't assume we, as a society, need to be walking spherical with N95 mask in our pockets for the rest of our lives. Figure out what is a good way of life alternate on your heath and the health of those round you. Then, determine out what are brief assets you'll do to reduce your threat of publicity. The pandemic hazard stages will alternate so that you can also even make a listing of adjustments and put into effect them primarily based completely totally on warning degree.

## Reactive vs Proactive

Think about the very last time you spilled a drink on a desk or counter. Sure, you may not were capable of get the preliminary splash but in the long run to procure some aspect to easy it up and raced to forestall it from spreading. Think about while you had the paper towels or towel on your hand, and also you were conducting out to prevent that one lengthy strip speeding its way towards some paper. When you thrust your hand out to wall it off, did you goal for in which it have become or a bit earlier of in which it became going to be at the same time as your hand have been given there.

THINK.

Likewise, whilst aiming to hit a transferring goal, do you aim for in which it is or in which it's miles going to be whilst the projectile meets it? Now undergo in mind a spill spreading in each course at random and you'll start to get an idea of the way a contagious disorder spreads. You need to head it off, you can't chase it.

You can't watch the records and tell yourself it's miles one u.S.A., or one county, or one metropolis away and also you don't want to worry approximately it. You can't take a look at humans as they get it, you can incredible affirm someone has it once they have had it and were spreading it for a while. Also, inside the present day age of excursion, the infectious disorder may be everywhere and spreading in a depend of hours.

You need to be way earlier of it.

This is why journey, big gatherings, and faculties is probably close down. It is an attempt to get ahead of it. Or, at the least, sluggish it down.

Behind the Power Curve in Preparedness

Unless you have your very very own survival retreat, live there and earn a living from home, have 7 years' properly absolutely well worth of food and water saved, have custom 4x4 vehicles that appear like some element out of GI Joe or Mad Max, then you definitely certainly're at the back of the power curve. That approach ninety nine.Nine% parents are behind the preparedness electricity curve. That kind of preparedness is a hard manner to stay and maximum people don't want to live it.

The proper news is that we're no longer probable looking at some thing near the apocalypse. Pandemics aren't an superb state of affairs through any stretch of the imagination, however it isn't the stop of the arena as we're aware of it. You don't have to shop for a ton of stuff that you'll by no means use. In my final "supply runs" I might also need to say 60% of what I supplied is stuff we will expend in the next month or so. Another 20% is stuff we're able to use every time we need, and it wouldn't be bizarre. Stuff like charcoal for the BBQ grill and paper plates.

Only 20% of the stuff I recommend, which you would probably buy, are things you'd possibly hide throwing your subsequent get collectively. I understand, you don't need people questioning you're bizarre or overreacting. Funny element is, they're hiding that stuff even as you return over too most probable.

Calm your fears, consciousness on what you're attempting to carry out, and execute. That's the manner you'll make it through an endemic simply excellent. You received't have many regrets if it seems to be much less than what you idea it is probably.


What if You Can't Prepare

If you're sick or disabled, you then definately're going to should rely upon your own family and pals. Find gentile strategies to speak your problems and your wishes. You don't need to feature any more stress to them in this already demanding event. At the same time, don't be so quiet and sacrificial that your situation receives worse. If your situation gets worse or then need to get you sources ultimate minute, you could turn out to be being more of a burden on the same time as seeking to be considerate. If you could't offer some thing else, offer emotional guide, statistics, and data.

Become their studies professional. If you're reading this ebook you aren't virtually vain.

If you've decided on to commit all your time and energy into selfish and useless endeavors, then you definately simply is probably out of achievement. If you're a diploma 1,000 wizard online, in case you're a legend at Call of Duty, if you're Instagram-Famous, if you're a liberal arts pupil, in case your existence is primarily based on uselessness and you haven't any coins, no abilities, no understanding of something beneficial, and if difficult paintings looks like torture, then your fantastic wager is probably to go to an emergency refuge and beg for them to can help you in.

I apprehend, "Never visit the Superdome." However, in case you're seen as now not whatever greater than a completely needy meals sucking doorstop, then why should genuinely absolutely everyone hazard themselves for you? Sometimes the herd desires to be thinned. I am not advocating that people shouldn't be charitable. To me, there is a super line with being charitable and sacrificing yourself due to the truth someone else have become silly. I do understand the selection to be merciful and assist others, but there can be also a call to make certain those with abilities, information, understanding, and proper art work ethics make it through a deadly disease. If all of the professional, hardworking, and clever die off in sacrificial love, all that is left in the back of may be idiots.

## Go Get Your Supplies Now

When I at the start wrote this phase, the Super Bowl had virtually finished, and the Impeachment became wrapping up. That wasn't that prolonged in the past. The worldwide has modified in only a few weeks with the cutting-edge pandemic. I'm leaving the specific phase in under as a memorial of kinds.

You need to be getting materials and gear now, if not months inside the past. Hopefully what you've got were given within the manner of meals, medical substances, and many others. The very last economic smash gives with resources so pass ahead and make a quick listing, do as a tremendous deal on line buying as you need to, after which come back to this phase.

Luckily, anyone has had the Super Bowl and Impeachment to focus on. Nobody is really paying attention to the REDACTED. Even in the occasion that they weren't distracted thru the modern-day hyped occasions, do you really expect they need to make the effort to tug themselves a protracted manner from their ordinary distractions? Most people see any diploma of preparedness as an overreaction and waste of time. They jokingly remind you of the Chicken-Little story and say, "The sky is falling!" Most human beings be troubled with the aid of what's known as Normalcy Bias.

Normalcy Bias is the perception humans preserve whilst there can be a excessive possibility of a catastrophe. It reasons people to underestimate every the probability of a catastrophe and its possible results, due to the fact human beings recall that matters will usually feature the manner things typically have functioned. It paralyzes them in a way that they may be nearly incapable of making geared up.

Think of storm season. It takes region every three hundred and sixty five days across the identical time. You may want to don't forget after going via 20 or 30 seasons, humans would will be inclined to hold some emergency substances to be had in regions that typically get hit the toughest. You need to even anticipate they could have elements available even as the hurricane is delivered and approximately 2 or three days out and absolutely everyone is going about their ordinary business organisation. But while the hurricane is 24 hours out, the shops turns into a madhouse and the cabinets are stripped bare.

Most humans don't be given as proper with some thing goes to reveal up until it's far barreling down on top of them. Most people don't famend a deadly disease till they for my part recognize a person who has died.

This in reality works in your desire in case you need to get additives at the very last minute in advance than anyone virtually realizes there can be a catastrophe. The keep shelves are usually full up until the last few days in advance than all hell breaks free. Take benefit of it.

These Will Build on One Another.

What I is probably recommending from right here on can be 3 degrees so that you can stack on every unique. Some might be starting to accumulate a few weeks of meals in diploma 3 after which in more food in tiers 2 and 1. The Level 3 listing is likely the largest list as it is the muse. It can also moreover have subjects that seem like not unusual revel in to some, however we'd all be amazed at what a few people don't apprehend or might likely need to be reminded of.

So, with that said, please be affected person and maintain reading in case you see something addressed in more than one phase. I will try and hold subjects that appear repetitive short and nice upload to it if vital.

It can be that you are probable beyond Level three by the time you get to look at this e-book. That doesn't make Level three any plenty a whole lot much less important. It is foundational.

Divide and Conquer

If you are dwelling with others, in case you are making plans and making ready with others, take some thing you find out beneficial in the coming sections and make a list. Divide that listing up and offer all of us some issue to do.

Some of these could in all likelihood encompass having the more youthful and further capable individuals of the family go out for belongings you could't find out on line. Some is probably discovering records. Everyone may also have to collect up their very personal data. This is lots to do.

Now, if you have participants of your corporation that don't accept as proper with in all of this preparedness and count on topics are in reality going to blow over in each week, then have them do some of the greater sensible duties which can be prudent for normal lifestyles. Have them address the car protection and round up the life insurance insurance records. They can recuperation the leaky faucet. They can take that vintage couch that's just taking up region to the unload. There are masses of things you can have them do that is virtually sensible things we might normally do or need to be doing. It might not be the maximum green branch of labor however getting them to do something is higher than no longer some thing.

Level three

As I stated, Level three is the foundation. From right here the whole thing is going up! This method you want to decide how far you could cross for your steering and handling a plague. I can't make that choice for you. Everyone has an opinion on how some distance to take it. But really as within the proactive instance, you need to be beforehand of this.

Level 3 is getting organized for a few element to show up. I apprehend some element can also need to already be going on as you have a look at this, however you might be in earlier stages than you observed. So, here you are getting subjects collectively and setting yourself up for "achievement" of sorts.

I take a look at preparedness as insurance. "How an entire lot am I inclined to pay to be prepared for X feasible scenario" is largely the query I ask myself. I weigh out how in all likelihood a scenario is and then how comfortable do I want to be if I have to stay thru it? There are lots of those who consider the information and don't think some thing will appear to them. I'm not a fortune teller so I can't say that some thing will appear to them. I can do math even though and I comprehend what the facts say.

So determine out for your self how a long way you're inclined to transport now, as you examine alongside. It will help you a fantastic deal in growing a plan and executing that pan.

Precaution Measures (Don't bypass the ones)

In guidance for coping with an endemic you want to get your house in order. There are some matters we need to reveal into conduct and some topics we want to get achieved. None of those ought to without a doubt be traumatic until you've got were given uncommon situations.

Clean up

Do your laundry and dishes. Vacuum and dirt. Take out the trash. Remove muddle. Google a way to smooth your property or rental. This is awesome essential. Clutter and disarray effect your capability to count on and attention. You want all your intellectual property

## Chapter 8: Make A Few Easy Plans And Percentage Them

Think through how you may do the standard responsibilities you take without any consideration in an emergency situation and make a plan B. Look, we're all hyper targeted on a plague inside the interim, but Mother Nature doesn't care. She will but ship awful weather our manner. It is regular to expect the energy going out in a storm. So, bear in thoughts how you could put together dinner without energy.

Any disruption to public utilities may be difficult to address if anyone is stuck at domestic. You can't truely call the constructing manager to get the house duties body of workers on it. You are the constructing supervisor and the house responsibilities frame of personnel most possibly. This isn't the apocalypse but just consider it, have a backup, and write it down.

Once you have a nicely concept out concept for a plan B, percentage it with a person who is like-minded or is aware of approximately it. Maybe an avid camper is probably useful? They is probably succesful to help you see a shortcoming in your plan you didn't take a look at. They also can benefit out of your concept and be capable of make themselves extra capable in an emergency.

Cooking

For most human beings, this is pretty smooth. If the power goes out, we get away the grill. If you've got a grill, make sure you have got sufficient gas. Don't burn garbage or paper because it is probably poisonous. If it is poisonous, it's going to contaminate the meals you eat and then you definately virtually have a new set of troubles. I without a doubt have a clean little charcoal grill and most of my cookware is chrome steel. That is my plan B. I'm not linking to a grill or grilling materials due to the reality all of them seem like obnoxiously highly-priced on Amazon. You can get one on Amazon, but I sincerely revel in responsible recommending it. It is probably safer than going to the store.

If you may skip get one then do not forget the extras like utensils. Just keep on with chrome steel and you'll be wonderful.

Apartment dwellers might have a tougher time.

I haven't used that model of hotplate, but it has right evaluations. I additionally admit that I actually have no longer researched using a batter and power inverter to run the ones sorts of domestic gadget. However, I apprehend a few humans who've. One individual honestly used a automobile battery and power inverter to hold their fridge going for walks and prepare dinner. Do some correct studies.

Disposable dinnerware

If you ever had to wash dishes thru manner of hand in a energy outage, inside the darkish, and in winter then you definately definitely definately recognise how depressing this is. I don't suppose all of us loves to do dishes. So, as to now not upload to my issues and devour more time with cleaning, I even have a deliver of paper plates and bowls at the aspect of plastic cups and plastic utensils.

I plan on using them for as many meals as I can. When I get about midway thru my stash, I will think about have turn out to be to preserve them. I want to be as unoccupied with chores as feasible whilst although staying on pinnacle of them. You don't need to reuse the ones due to the truth foodborne bacteria begins growing as rapid as the meals hits the plate and cools down.

Fire prevention

If I'm mentioning cooking, then it is a exquisite time to say fireplace safety. Buy a fire extinguisher for any area that is more likely to make fireplace, like kitchens. Have a further one to hold outside in case you're grilling close to your house.

I assume a well-known ABC fireside extinguisher works brilliant for ordinary domestic uses. Call your neighborhood fireplace department in case you don't understand a bargain about them. I'm sure they might be satisfied to help you. If they aren't willing to help you, remind them that hearth prevention is truly honestly considered one of their mandates and that they art work for the citizens and residents in their place. Do it in a polite manner. Also ask if they might provide you with and your family an indication. It is good to apprehend the way to use one BEFORE you need to understand the manner to use one.

I use a few considered one of a type sizes of ABC extinguishers relying on in which I am storing it and the dimensions of fireplace it is probably used to assist extinguish. I use a few problem similar to this 5lb ABC Dry Chemical Fire Extinguisher, Amazon Link: https://amzn.To/2Qg3csl

It is likewise an superb time to vicinity new batteries on your smoke detectors and any other tracking tool you have got were given.

Waste manipulate

Luckily, while strength goes out most bathrooms keep flushing. If which have been to prevent, it might be a crappy scenario (pun supposed). I'm now not an professional in sanitation but my plan B is the Luggable Loo Portable 5 Gallon Toilet, Amazon

It's no longer a long-term solution however I don't foresee us wanting a long-term answer. I plan on the usage of this, contractor grade trash baggage, and clumping kitty litter. I could probably located a small layer of kitty muddle on the lowest and clearly cover the mess because it takes place. I wouldn't allow it get too high.

Toilet Paper Shortage

People can also additionally need to have made a run at the relaxation room paper and maximum humans ought to probably then have a hard time finding any. In reaction human beings might be presenting up answers that seem a piece unsanitary. They variety from entering into direct contact with feces and then washing or using reusable cloths. I recognize that in greater rugged situations, you need to do what you have to do.

Industrial vendors promote relaxation room paper for public restrooms under particular names. You can generally find some component similar to the Morcon Paper 29 Millennium Bath Tissue after the crazies have bought the whole lot else up, Amazon link: https://amzn.To/39BBsW1

My compromise could be to use non flushable products like tissues or moist napkins and then take away them in a trash can for diapers as they've a seal typically. The P Playtex Diaper Genie Baby Registry Gift Set has everything you need,

There is task with fecal borne illnesses so carry out a piece homework and keep the entirety as smooth as feasible.

Trash

You won't deliver it a bargain perception, but the trash elimination provider is a massive part of our everyday lives. If that is interrupted, existence will cope with new dangers and a modern-day aroma. If the trash piles up on the reduce too prolonged, then three subjects take place:

- Bacteria grows in all the herbal trash and has the opportunity of spreading sickness.

- It will trap animals. These animals will not handiest make a large variety, however they will pose a hazard counting on your nearby natural worldwide.

- It will make your network heady scent horrible in an effort to kill morale.

I don't understand what is criminal right right here, however I plan on burning paper trash if possible. I don't endorse the usage of it as fuel for a few trouble. I will burn it to reduce the trash I will set out at the size down. I became planning on the usage of my grill as a burn barrel on the same time as now not the use of it to cook dinner and dumping the ash in trash baggage destined for the reduce down. You can find out burn barrels on Amazon, but I don't realise enough approximately them to advocate any.

An exciting despite the fact that, if you use sawdust for your emergency rest room then it is probably feasible to burn the human waste and trash on the equal time. Please research this as I assume I actually have observe approximately long time illnesses from inhaling those fumes, however I am not fine.

Communication

During the Sept. 11 assault, phones strains had been jammed for a huge part of the day with human beings calling round looking for their cherished ones. The infrastructure isn't designed to have all of us calling on the identical time. The infrastructure is also energy based. So it is continually accurate to have a plan B.

While the cellphone lines is probably tied up, the net need to regardless of the reality that be running. Texting is ideal for brief messages, but it isn't first rate for conveying something more complicated. I recommend locating out a few difficulty like Skype, a few different Voice Over Internet Protocol (VOIP), or video messaging as those are net bandwidth based totally. If all people is hogging the bandwidth, attempt minimizing what you need through the usage of actually voice features.

www.ingramcontent.com/pod-product-compliance
Lightning Source LLC
Chambersburg PA
CBHW060501030426
42337CB00015B/1676